EMPOWER YOURSELF

Latest, Greatest Speed Cures from Today's Top Doctors

Hidden Healthcare Dangers and Rip-Offs

Doctor-Tested Home Remedies for Everything
from Hiccups to Hemorrhoids

Keep Your Mind Razor-Sharp for Life!

The New Super Foods for Super Health!

Fast Fixes for Stubborn Health Problems

Color Away Your Anxiety and Stress!

Throw Away Your Diabetes Medications!

Have the Best Sex of Your Life After 60!

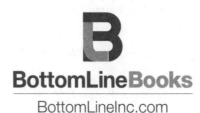

BottomLineBooks

BottomLineInc.com

First printing

Bottom Line Books® is a registered trademark of Bottom Line Inc.
3 Landmark Square, Suite 201, Stamford, CT 06901

www.bottomlineinc.com

Bottom Line Books is an imprint of Bottom Line Inc., publisher of print periodicals, e-letters and books. We are dedicated to bringing you the best information from the most knowledgeable sources in the world. Our goal is to help you gain greater wealth, better health, more wisdom, extra time and increased happiness.

Printed in the United States of America

SHL/am

Contents

Contents

1

Latest, Greatest Speed Cures from Today's Top Doctors

Breakthrough Cancer Treatment

It seems like every week there's a promising new cancer treatment—that never happens. Too often we read about a new theoretical approach that saves lives in one or two studies...only to wait and wait for the treatment to materialize in the practice of cancer medicine. This time is different.

Now the powerful cancer-fighting drugs are not theoretical or another case of overhyping, overpromising and underdelivering. These medications really do work. This new way of fighting cancer uses the body's own immune system to wage war on cancer cells. Many leading cancer experts believe this approach, known as cancer immunotherapy, could revolutionize how we treat many forms of cancer.

When it comes to certain cancers, the revolution has already begun. In fact, former president Jimmy Carter is now said to be "cancer free" (based on MRI scans) after using one of these drugs for the melanoma that spread to his brain.

The new treatments aren't about enhancing immunity in general. Instead, this is an intriguing approach that can prevent cancerous tumors from hijacking our own immune defenses—so that our amazing immune system can do its job.

6 THINGS YOU NEED TO KNOW

Here are the details on this latest form of cancer immunotherapy...

1. It treats the body's immune system so the immune system can fight the cancer. T cells are the immune system's main line of defense, but they're not always effective against cancer cells. In the 1990s, cancer researchers identified a class of molecules in the body that are known as immune checkpoints. These molecules keep T cells from attacking

---

Louis Weiner, MD, director, Lombardi Comprehensive Cancer Center, Georgetown University, Washington, DC. He is an internationally recognized medical oncologist specializing in the treatment of gastrointestinal cancers. His lab researches novel immunotherapy treatments.

1

normal cells, but cancer cells can hijack them for their own purposes. Cancer cells employ immune "checkpoints" to turn off killer T cells that would otherwise recognize and destroy a cancer that was growing in a person's body. Drugs that block these checkpoints so T cells can do their job are game changers called immune checkpoint inhibitors.

2. It still has side effects, but early results suggest a less toxic experience. All of us would love to see a day when very toxic chemotherapy agents that cause hair loss, low blood counts, fatigue, etc., are no longer the backbone of therapy for cancer. With checkpoint inhibitors, there will potentially be fewer side effects and certainly different ones. So far, the most common side effects caused by checkpoint inhibitors already in use include fatigue, cough, nausea, skin rash and itching. But more serious side effects including severe diarrhea, colitis and intestinal inflammation (even perforation) have also been reported.

3. It can be very effective and long-lasting. Consider the effects of checkpoint inhibitors against end-stage Hodgkin's disease, where patients had already received every imaginable therapy and were running out of hope. More than 90% of these patients went into remissions, many of them complete. When checkpoint inhibitors are combined against metastatic melanoma—the most deadly form of skin cancer—more than half of those cancers are eliminated or controlled, with benefits that have lasted for many years in some cases.

4. It works against many forms of cancer. In a viewpoint recently published in *JAMA*, James Allison, PhD, who pioneered the use of immune checkpoint inhibitors against cancer, wrote: "The therapy does not target the tumor cell but rather engages a target on the patient's immune system. Thus, there is no inherent reason that it would not be successful against a wide variety of tumors."

At this time, checkpoint inhibitors are FDA approved for treating only certain types of melanoma and lung cancer. But studies show that they also work against no fewer than 20 different cancers, including certain forms of kidney cancer, triple negative breast cancer, stomach cancer, Hodgkin's disease, bladder cancer and head and neck cancer.

5. It is very expensive. It can cost tens of thousands of dollars or more to have a course of therapy with these drugs, especially if you start combining them with other expensive cancer therapies.

6. It is still evolving. One promising innovation in cancer immunotherapy that is currently being researched is chimeric antigen receptor (CAR) T-cell therapy. In this case, a patient's T cells are genetically engineered to produce antibodies against a specific type of cancer. When these T cells proliferate, they pass their cancer-killing modifications along.

So far, this experimental treatment has had outstanding results against a hard-to-treat and deadly form of leukemia called acute lymphocytic leukemia.

WHAT'S AVAILABLE NOW

While many checkpoint inhibitors are in development, currently only three have been approved by the FDA…

• **Opdivo** (*nivolumab*) and **Keytruda** (*pembrolizumab*) are approved for advanced-stage non-small cell lung cancer that has spread and that is not responding to conventional platinum-based chemotherapy…and for advanced melanoma.

• **Yervoy** (*ipilimumab*) is approved for melanoma that has spread within the body (metastasized) or that cannot be removed by surgery.

Until new drugs for different cancers make it through the FDA approval process—or the existing approved ones get future approvals for different cancers—these are the only three of this type of cancer treatment that insurance companies or Medicare are likely to cover. If you have the financial wherewithal, you may be able to have your doctor prescribe the approved drugs off-label and pay for them yourself.

For everyone else, however, there is another potential option. If there is an immunotherapy cancer drug in development for a cancer that you are being treated for, ask your oncologist whether there is a clinical trial that you can join. You can also check the website *Clinical Trials.gov.*

High-Intensity Focused Ultrasound for Prostate Cancer

Thomas Gardner, MD, associate professor of urology at Indiana University School/ of Medicine in Indianapolis, Indiana. Dr. Gardner specializes in the care of patients with cancers of the urinary system including prostate, kidney and bladder.

S ome men with prostate cancer are planning expensive trips abroad—but not for vacation. They are seeking a high-tech and somewhat controversial treatment for their cancer that promises fewer side effects and a rapid recovery—and, perhaps, higher odds of survival. Only recently approved by the FDA here in the US for prostate cancer, the minimally invasive HIFU (High Intensity Focused Ultrasound) uses focused ultrasound beams to heat the prostate to temperatures higher than 80 degrees Celsius, destroying cancer cells. While it sounds promising, this procedure is not as simple as it first appears to be. There are risks inherent to traveling abroad for medical procedures, in general. *And then there's the treatment itself…*

AN UNFINISHED TALE

HIFU treats prostate cancer without destroying surrounding tissue, reducing the likelihood of problems such as incontinence and impotence, which are often associated with other treatments such as surgery, radiation and cryotherapy. This is alluring to the growing number of prostate cancer patients who, expecting to live years beyond their treatment, want to preserve their health and quality of life. Though one in six American men will be diagnosed with the disease in their lifetime, only one in 35 will die from it.

HIFU can be an excellent technology when used "in the right hands among appropriate patients," according to Thomas Gardner, MD, associate professor of urology at Indiana University School of Medicine in Indianapolis. He is a researcher involved in clinical trials of Sonablate HIFU here in the US. Phase I/II trial results, published in the *Journal of Urology* in December 2007, were encouraging: "High-intensity focused ultrasound in patients with previously untreated prostate cancer is generally well tolerated and it has the potential to completely ablate the prostate gland," their study concluded, noting "with further refinement of the optimal treatment dose and technique, this technology has the potential to be an effective form of therapy for localized prostate cancer." However, research efforts have been partly delayed for the Phase III trial due to recruitment and funding problems.

Of course, given risks of the current treatment options, such as surgery, many men are still anxious to try what appears to be a better, more tolerable and more effective method. Though there are claims of fewer side effects compared with other prostate cancer treatments, Dr. Gardner said this has yet to be proven—and the same holds true for HIFU's long-term cure rates. No published US clinical trial data comparing long-term cure rates of HIFU with other standard prostate cancer therapies is available.

HOW HIFU WORKS

There are two types of HIFU technologies, neither approved in the US. Both use a transrectal probe to deliver ultrasound energy directly to the prostate without causing damage to areas outside of the gland. "This technology can spare nerves, whereas other prostate cancer treatments often cannot," Dr. Gardner explained.

• **Sonablate.** This technology is available in Mexico as well as Canada, the Dominican Republic, Costa Rica, Argentina, Japan, Europe, South Africa…and now in the US. The equipment uses a split-beam technology allowing the doctor to visualize and treat the cancerous area. It has four different probes of varying focal lengths that can all be used sequentially in one treatment session. "The Sonablate is a more controllable device because it can provide adjustable focused ultrasound," explained Dr. Gardner. HIFU with Sonablate is an outpatient procedure usually lasting between two and three hours, depending on the size of the prostate. Since it involves no incision, cutting or radiation, it can easily be repeated if necessary. It can also be used as a salvage therapy if there is a recurrence of cancer in the event other treatments fail.

•**Ablatherm.** In comparison, this is a device produced by the French company EDAP TMS and is approved for use in Canada, Europe, Russia, South Korea and Australia. It employs just a single focal zone length and does not allow for monitoring during treatment. It's more of a "'one size fits all' device because it only delivers focused ultrasound at one distance," says Dr. Gardner. Also, Ablatherm sometimes requires a pre-surgical procedure, called a transurethral resection of the prostate (TURP) in large prostates, while the Sonablate does not.

THE PRICE IS ONE BIG PROBLEM

Beyond a lack of data, the real downside of HIFU for consumers is cost. Treatment can range between $10,000 and $25,000, depending on where the patient is treated. Insurance companies rarely pick up the tab. It's perhaps understandable that some patients, especially those with deep pockets, might waive those concerns, but the problem with seeking HIFU treatment overseas is that some clinics offering the therapy may be largely motivated by big profits, says Dr. Gardner, not quality patient care. The results can be devastating. Many off-shore sites seek to treat as many patients as quickly as they can… potentially leaving a significant percentage under-treated. Due to the size of the prostate and amount of time it takes to treat it effectively, two or three HIFU treatments may be required to eradicate the cancer—and patients are not necessarily told this before they begin.

For prostate cancer patients who are nonetheless interested in pursuing HIFU, how can they protect themselves?

First, says Dr. Gardner, is to find out whether or not it's a good therapy for their cancer. HIFU therapy is reasonable for patients who meet all these criteria:

•**Early stage (T1 or T2) cancer** with localized (organ-confined) tumors

•**A Gleason score** (a grading score of the prostate tumor that indicates how likely the tumor is to spread) of less than or equal to 6

•**A PSA level less than 10 ng/mL**

•**Have had a recent (within six months) prostate biopsy that is positive for cancer cells.**

•**A prostate volume of less than 40 cc.**

Be sure to carefully investigate the quality of physicians and facilities at the HIFU clinic you are considering. Dr. Gardner has concerns about the treatments in certain foreign countries, where he believes there's not as much control over the quality of care.

FDA approval of HIFU in the US has made a vital option available for prostate cancer patients. However, Dr. Gardner urges caution. "Patients should be very careful," he said. "There are several established techniques, such as surgery, radiation and cryotherapy, available in the US for the treatment of localized prostate cancer. While these do have some risk to future male function, unlike HIFU, they are generally conducted in approved hospital or surgical settings." Patients need to be aware of the inevitable learning curve surrounding this relatively new treatment on US soil.

Do not sign up for treatment unless you have thoroughly discussed your case and your eligibility with your doctor, he cautions.

New Prostate Cancer Test

The Prostate Health Index (PHI), a new blood test, is three times more accurate than the prostate-specific antigen (PSA) test. Because the protein that is measured by the PSA test can be elevated due to prostate cancer—or prostate inflammation or enlargement—this test often leads to unnecessary biopsies.

Now: The PHI test, which analyzes three different protein markers, was found to be more accurate and reduced the need for unnecessary biopsies by 31%.

William J. Catalona, MD, director, Clinical Prostate Cancer Program, Robert H. Lurie Comprehensive Cancer Center of Northwestern University, Chicago.

body) with pressure that is firm but not painful. After a session, your skin should be slightly pink. If it's red or irritated, you're pressing too hard. Each session should last five to 10 minutes. Do it twice a day to keep your lymphatic system functioning efficiently.

●**Self-massage.** Some massage therapists are trained in lymphatic drainage massage. Professional treatments are a good choice for patients with lymphedema, swelling that may occur after a mastectomy or other cancer treatments. But for less serious lymphatic congestion, self-massage works just as well.

What to do: Very lightly stroke the congested area, slowly moving your fingers at least a few inches from the affected area toward your heart for a few minutes. If you are coming down with a cold, for example, gently stroke swollen lymph nodes every few hours.

●**Pokeweed salve/liquid.** I often prescribe this herbal therapy for patients with hard or tender lymph nodes due to inflammation/infection. The active ingredients are transported through the skin and act as a lymphatic solvent. Improvement usually occurs within a few days. It's typically applied two to three times daily for two weeks.

Pokeweed is available at most health-food stores, but I advise using it only under the supervision of a doctor who specializes in herbal remedies. The herb contains alkaloid compounds that can potentially cause serious side effects, including changes in heart rate and/or difficulty breathing. People with kidney disease or other chronic conditions should not use pokeweed.

●**More water.** If you're dehydrated, the kidneys are less able to filter and eliminate wastes. Buildups of cellular by-products thicken lymph and impair normal circulation. The usual advice is to drink eight glasses of water a day, but some people need more—or less. One way to ensure proper hydration is to check your urine to see if it is pale yellow.

For a more accurate assessment: Buy a pack of urine dipsticks. They are inexpensive and sold at pharmacies with indicators to check specific gravity, a measure of urine concentration. If you're drinking enough water according to the specific gravity reading (ask your health-care provider for your optimal reading), use the dipstick once a week. Otherwise, use it daily until your hydration status improves.

The Hidden Vitamin Deficiency

Patrick C. J. Ward, MD, a professor emeritus of biomedical sciences and former chair of the department of anatomy, microbiology and pathology at the University of Minnesota Medical School in Duluth.

Most people are familiar with "iron poor blood." But there's another deficiency that's less well-known—one that can cause a variety of troubling symptoms and occurs even when people do their best to eat a healthful diet. Vitamin B-12 levels that are lower than normal can be associated with muscle weakness, fatigue and/or memory problems. More severe deficiencies can cause irreversible nerve damage...or be a factor in premature death.

EASY TO MISS

The initial symptoms of low B-12 (mentioned above) can be caused by many unrelated conditions, including hypothyroidism and depression. And because older adults are the ones most likely to suffer from B-12 deficiencies, their complaints might be dismissed as normal age-related problems.

What's more: Most doctors diagnose B-12 anemia (lack of healthy red blood cells due to a B-12 deficiency) only when levels fall below about 200 picograms per milliliter (pg/mL) of blood serum. But older people with higher levels of B-12 can still experience symptoms.

WHO SHOULD GET TESTED

If you have any of the symptoms above—or if a routine blood test uncovers certain abnormalities (see below)—ask your doctor to test you for B-12 anemia. *Who's at risk...*

●**Adults age 50 and older.** The age-related drop in pepsin and other digestive fluids can impair the body's ability to absorb B-12. The same thing can happen in those who regularly take acid-suppressing heartburn drugs, such as *esomeprazole* (Nexium) or *omeprazole* (Prilosec).

• **Strict vegetarians and vegans.** With the exception of fortified foods (such as breakfast cereals) and supplements, animal products (meat, fish, dairy, eggs, etc.) are the only sources of vitamin B-12.

• **People with pernicious anemia.** About 1% to 2% of older adults have pernicious anemia, a form of B-12 anemia caused by an autoimmune disorder in which the body cannot absorb adequate levels of B-12 to make enough red blood cells. Your doctor might suspect this if you have symptoms of B-12 deficiency or if a blood test shows abnormal blood cells (see below).

• **Anyone with macrocytosis, or enlarged red blood cells.** This condition is one of the first signs of a B-12 deficiency. It's often discovered during blood tests performed for a routine physical or for conditions such as peripheral neuropathy.

FIRST-LINE TESTING

The first test a doctor will order if he/she suspects a B-12 deficiency is a complete blood count (CBC), which is included in many routine checkups. Among other things, the test will show your mean corpuscular volume (MCV), the average size of red blood cells. If you have a B-12 deficiency, the red cells will usually be larger than normal. You'll also have lower-than-expected hemoglobin (an iron-rich protein that helps carry oxygen/carbon dioxide) and hematocrit (the percentage of blood consisting of red blood cells).

However: High MCV won't prove that you have a deficiency. The same results can be caused by other conditions, such as heavy alcohol use, folate deficiency or a precursor to leukemia. But it does alert your doctor that low B-12 is a possibility. High MCV requires further testing for B-12 and/or folate deficiency. A blood smear that shows the presence of at least one six-lobed neutrophil (white blood cell) strongly indicates a B-12 and/or folate deficiency.

You'd think that the easiest way to detect a B-12 deficiency would be to simply measure B-12, also known as cobalamin, in the blood.

Many doctors who check their patients' B-12 levels like the serum cobalamin test because it's an inexpensive starting point (about $100 and usually covered by insurance).

If your level of B-12 is solidly in the normal range (350 pg/mL or above), you probably won't need any other tests for B-12. But it's not the best test in some cases. Why? The results of this test can be somewhat misleading—for instance, levels are falsely low in at least 20% of cases.

Also: Many people who have this test will be told that their B-12 is "low-normal"—a gray zone between 200 pg/mL and 350 pg/mL. The word "normal" means that they won't be diagnosed with a deficiency...and might continue to suffer from symptoms of B-12 deficiency.

DEFINITIVE TESTS

If your symptoms still suggest a B-12 deficiency but the tests are not definitive, your doctor may want to take testing to another level. To do this, he will order a blocking antibody test to look for antibodies that render intrinsic factor (a protein needed to promote B-12 absorption) ineffective. A positive test indicates autoimmune B-12 deficiency (pernicious anemia). You can easily be treated for it (see below) and will require no further testing.

If the diagnosis is still uncertain, a fairly definitive test for B-12 deficiency is a methylmalonic acid (MMA) test. B-12 is needed for MMA to break down fatty acids. But if B-12 is inadequate, more MMA will accumulate. One study found that 98.4% of those with elevated MMA had B-12 levels under 200 pg/mL. This test is somewhat expensive (about $200) and not always covered by insurance.

EASY TO TREAT

Although a deficiency of B-12 can cause many troubling symptoms or even serious health problems, it's also among the easiest of conditions to prevent—and treat.

The Institute of Medicine advises adults to get 2.4 micrograms (mcg) of vitamin B-12 daily from meat and other animal foods or from fortified foods, such as breakfast cereals. A three-ounce serving of salmon has 4.8 mcg... one cup of low-fat milk has 1.2 mcg...and a serving of fortified cereal has at least 1.5 mcg.

If you've tested low, you'll probably need B-12 injections. They're usually given in a doctor's office or they can be self-injected once a week for eight weeks, then monthly thereafter. Patients with pernicious anemia or other conditions that impair B-12 absorption will need the injections for life. Others may be able to stop the injections once normal B-12 levels are restored.

Research has shown that oral B-12 supplements can be as effective as injections. The starting dose for a supplement is 2 mg daily... and is then lowered to 1 mg daily, then weekly and, finally, monthly.

A Quick-Step Fecal Transplant Pill For C. Diff Diarrhea

Eamonn Quigley, MBBS, MD, chief, division of gastroenterology and hepatology and medical director at The Lynda K. and David M. Underwood Center for Digestive Disorders, The Methodist Hospital and Weill Cornell College of Medicine, Houston.

You may have heard of a gross but highly effective technique for treating certain gut problems—namely Clostridium difficile infection, a common cause of chronic diarrhea and stomach upset in people older than 65, people who have been on antibiotics for a long time and people whose immune systems are down, such as cancer patients. The treatment, called fecal transplantation, involves taking purified feces from a healthy person and putting it into a sick one.

Known to Chinese medicine and other non-Western forms of healing for thousands of years, fecal transplant took the medical community by storm when Western doctors realized that it really worked—and so much better than pharma drugs. The cure rate for chronic C. difficile infection treated with fecal transplant is about 90%. In fact, doctors were so impressed with the success of fecal transplants that they negotiated, in full force, with the FDA when the FDA threatened to put tight restrictions on when and how the procedure could be performed.

STREAMLINING FECAL TRANSPLANTS

The point of fecal transplants is to transfer healthful gut bacteria (found in healthy human feces) from one person into another so that these bacteria can populate that other person's gut and edge out the microbes and chemical reactions that are causing disease, explained Eamonn Quigley, MBBS, MD, an expert in fecal transplant and chief of the division of gastroenterology and hepatology at The Methodist Hospital and Weill Cornell Medical College in Houston. In ancient China—brace yourself—transplants were performed by feeding a person "poop soup." Nowadays, fecal transplants are performed via enema or by inserting a tube into the colon or the stomach through the nose. But there's got to be a better way—and that way is soon to debut—a way most Americans are, ironically, used to when it comes to treating infections. A pill. But not a pill loaded with synthetic drugs. This pill contains frozen or freeze-dried human feces.

Scientists have been experimenting with this treatment since 2013 and, most recently, a research team from the Massachusetts General Hospital proved that fecal transplant pills work as well as the more invasive methods just mentioned. The team recruited 20 patients with chronic C. difficile infections and gave them pills containing freeze-dried stool (screened for safety) donated by volunteers. Each patient took 15 capsules a day for two days. And even though that still sounds gross, the treatment worked like a charm. Diarrhea stopped and did not return in 14 of the 20 patients (70%). The six patients who still had symptoms got another two-day treatment a week later, and five were cured (although C. difficile symptoms recurred after a few weeks in one of the five who responded to the second treatment). That means that the fecal pill was 90% successful. These folks would otherwise have been treated with heavy-duty and expensive antibiotics, such as vancomycin and metronidazole—antibiotics that can have side effects and often don't work anyway.

WHO NEEDS IT?

Do a search of fecal transplants on the Web and you will learn that some people are advocating at-home, do-it-yourself fecal transplants. But do-it-yourself jobs are risky…instead of curing an infection, you could give yourself one from parasites and bad bacteria lurking in your donor's feces, or you could infect or injure yourself from homespun methods of getting the feces into yourself, said Dr. Quigley. As for medically done procedures, no cases of serious side effects have been reported.

Although fecal transplant might be useful for other gut infections and even chronic illnesses such as inflammatory bowel disease, it is now approved only to treat C. difficile infections. The pill form of fecal transplant continues to be studied and isn't yet officially ready for prime time, but the odds seem very good that the pill method will soon be approved, given the dramatic results of the latest study.

If you have C. difficile infection and have been bombarding your body with antibiotics for it because the infection keeps coming back, visit a gastroenterologist and ask about fecal transplant or visit *TheFecalTransplant Foundation.org* for gastroenterologists in your area who offer the treatment.

You Need Exercise—Not a Knee Replacement

Mitchell Yass, DPT, founder and director of PT2 Physical Therapy and Personal Training. He is the author of *Overpower Pain: The Strength-Training Program that Stops Pain without Drugs or Surgery.* MitchellYass.com

---

Did you know that knee-replacement surgery is virtually epidemic in this country? The number has doubled over the past decade. And among Medicare beneficiaries, the number of knee replacements has increased by more than 160%. One recent research paper reported that 4 million Americans now have knee implants—including half a million who had to have their knee replacement redone at least once. What explains all the extra knee replacements?

It's hard not to suspect that a lot of unnecessary operations are being done. *Here are the things you must know before letting someone cut out your knee…*

KNEE-REPLACEMENT RAMPAGE

A recent study showed that just about one-third of all knee replacements are inappropriate. The patients had relatively low levels of pain that could have been managed in other ways, and/or their knee X-rays showed little evidence of substantial arthritic changes. Many patients who were inappropriately given knee replacements were under age 55, and for them, considering that the life expectancy of the artificial joint is 15 to 20 years, another—and then perhaps another—arduous replacement operation will be needed.

Why are so many people so willingly getting an operation that is expensive, can take a year for full recovery and is certainly not without serious risks, including deadly blood clots? Mitchell Yass, DPT, the founder and owner of PT2 Physical Therapy and Personal Training, is a leading authority on physical therapy and an outspoken critic of overdiagnosis and misdiagnosis of musculoskeletal pain. According to Yass, most patients—and their doctors—jump to the conclusion that they need a knee replacement because of pain due to arthritis, but pain is not a reason for knee replacement or necessarily a sign of knee arthritis.

Studies that have looked at pain in relation to arthritic changes have shown that only about 15% of people with X-ray evidence of knee arthritis actually have knee pain. One study even showed that sham surgery relieved knee pain caused by osteoarthritis just as well as real surgery. "Clearly the relationship between osteoarthritis and knee pain cannot be directly correlated," said Yass.

THE REAL CAUSE OF KNEE PAIN

"Most people who suffer knee pain experience the pain around the kneecap. The pain is caused by an imbalance in the strength of the quadriceps muscles on the front of the thigh and the hamstring muscle on the back of it. The quadriceps naturally get a lot more use from walking and everyday activity and naturally tend to be much stronger than the hamstrings," Yass said. When the hamstring muscles are weaker than the quads, the quads shorten. This increases tension on the knee-cap. Instead of painlessly gliding along with the joint, the kneecap presses against the joint…painfully.

Another possible, but less likely, cause of knee pain, Yass said, is either a strain on the quadriceps or the band of connective tissue that runs from the hip to the outer side of the kneecap (called the iliotibial band). Strain on the quads will cause the kneecap to "float" outward, and strain on the iliotibial band will cause the knee cap to edge toward the left or right side of the knee joint. Either way, when the knee bends or straightens, the kneecap rubs against points in the knee joint that it shouldn't, causing pain.

THE REAL SOLUTION

"Joints are nothing more than 'pivot points' that exist solely to allow range of motion," Yass said. "When a joint has undergone arthritic changes severe enough to prevent motion, then and only then is surgery warranted." To be sure, there are people whose knees have been so degraded by wear and tear that replacement is the only current option to provide them with normal use of their knee. But Yass suggests that those people are actually rather few and far between. Rather than knee-replacement surgery, most people with knee pain need exercise to keep leg and knee muscles balanced and toned.

If you have knee pain, consider trying the exercises on the next page to improve and balance your leg muscles and avoid the type of knee symptoms that have convinced too many people—and their doctors—that they need knee-replacement surgery. (Do check with your doctor first—but there is seldom a good medical reason not to try exercises before going to surgery.) How many reps should you do? Do each exercise 10 times, take a one-minute break, then repeat two more sets. How frequently? Two or three times a week.

•**Loosen the Quads.** Stand near a wall for support. If your left knee is the most bothersome, turn your right side to the wall and rest your right hand against it. Then, reach back with your left hand to grip your left foot or

ankle. Gently pull the foot toward the buttocks until you feel a stretch in the front of your thigh. Hold for about 20 to 30 seconds. Repeat on the other side whether or not you have problems with the other knee to keep all the muscles in balance.

•**Strengthen the Hamstrings.** Practice the straight leg dead lift. To do this, stand with your legs hip width apart, hands at hip level either holding hand weights or grasping a pole (such a broomstick) horizontally in front of you. Bend forward from your hips, keeping your legs straight (without "locking" your knees) and letting your hands (holding weights or a pole) run down your thighs until you begin to feel a pull at the back of the thighs. Then immediately return to the start position. Do three sets of 10 repetitions.

•**Strengthen the Calves.** In Yass's experience, strengthening the calves can help offset excessive tightening of the quads and can strengthen the hamstrings. To do this exercise, stand facing a wall, counter or sturdy chair and place both hands on it to keep your balance. Rise up onto the balls of the feet (lifting your heels)…then, gently lower your heels to the ground. Once you feel that you can keep your balance when doing this exercise, you can hold dumbbells, which will create more muscle resistance and help strengthen the calves even more.

By the third week of doing these exercises, you should notice a significant improvement, said Yass. But even if you are completely rid of pain, you ought to keep up your exercise routine to keep the pain from returning. "You have to keep your muscles strong your entire life to keep them functional," said Yass. "It's like brushing your teeth to keep decay away."

Yoga Fights Pain

Chronic pain sufferers should hit the yoga mat, we hear from M. Catherine Bushnell, PhD. Chronic pain can cause loss of gray matter in the brain, which can lead to memory loss, cognitive impairment, emotional problems and reduced pain tolerance.

Recent finding: Practicing yoga can actually increase gray matter in the brain, including in the area related to pain tolerance.

M. Catherine Bushnell, PhD, scientific director, National Center for Complementary and Integrative Health, Bethesda, Maryland.

When Shoulder Pain Won't Go Away

Beth E. Shubin Stein, MD, an associate attending orthopedic surgeon and a member of the Sports Medicine and Shoulder Service at the Hospital for Special Surgery in New York City.

When you've got a painful shoulder, you're reminded of it many times each day. It can hurt when you're, say, scratching your back, taking off your shirt or washing your hair. If it's severe, the pain can even wake you up at night.

As many as half of all Americans suffer from shoulder pain each year. For a significant number of these people, the problem lingers on… for weeks, months or even longer.

There is hope: Whether the pain stems from an injury, overuse or some unknown cause, chronic shoulder pain can be dramatically improved—and usually eliminated. The treatments may also help those whose shoulder pain is caused by arthritis. *Here are the latest approaches for the most common shoulder problems…*

ROTATOR CUFF PROBLEMS

Most people are quick to chalk up shoulder pain to tendinitis, a nagging form of inflammation. But that's usually a mistake.

Recent thinking: The shoulder pain thought of as tendinitis is typically a result of tendinosis, a related condition that occurs when the tendons (ropelike cords connecting muscle to bone) begin to deteriorate. Tendinosis can usually be diagnosed with a physical exam and an X-ray and/or MRI.

Red flag for the patient: The pain may be barely perceptible while the arm is at rest—but if you extend the arm outward, in front of the body or overhead, the pain can range from dull to excruciating.

Rotator cuff tendinosis develops when tendons in the rotator cuff (a group of tendons and muscles that attach the upper arm to the shoulder joint) break down over time. This can occur due to age…repetitive use…or weakness of the rotator cuff muscles.

What works best: During the first week or two, to "quiet" the inflammation around the tendon, apply ice (for 15 to 20 minutes several times daily)…and take a nonsteroidal anti-inflammatory drug (NSAID), such as *ibuprofen* (Motrin).

If pain continues, your doctor should also refer you to a physical or occupational therapist, who can recommend exercises (such as those on the next page) to strengthen the rotator cuff and shoulder blade (scapula) muscles. If pain worsens or lasts longer than a week or two, a cortisone injection into the bursa surrounding the rotator cuff tendons can help.

Good news: Within six weeks, this nonsurgical regimen alleviates the pain 90% of the time.

Beware: Chronic use of cortisone can damage tendons, so surgery (see below) should be considered if two or three injections (given no more than every three months) have not relieved the pain.

If you don't get relief after six weeks or the pain returns after cortisone therapy wears off, you may want to consider surgery. Arthroscopy (inserting a tiny camera via small incisions) allows the surgeon to assess the shoulder joint and correct the damage that has led to rotator cuff tendinosis. When performed by an experienced surgeon, the procedure has a high success rate. Complications are rare but may involve infection or stiffness.

To find an experienced surgeon, consult The American Orthopaedic Society for Sports Medicine, *SportsMed.org.*

Two approaches that are less invasive than surgery…

•**Platelet-rich plasma (PRP) injection involves the use of platelets from a patient's blood.** The platelets are separated from the blood with a centrifuge and reinfused into the affected tendons. The platelets are rich in growth factors that aid healing, and the technique is considered safe, since the patient's own cells are used.

A small study published in 2013 in *Global Advances in Health and Medicine* found that a single PRP injection significantly improved pain and function at a 12-week follow-up. More research is needed, however, for definitive evidence of its effectiveness. Some patients opt to have a series of PRP injections. Insurance rarely covers the cost—typically about $1,500 per injection.

•**Stem cell treatment.** With this therapy, which is currently experimental, certain bone marrow cells are reinjected into the shoulder area, where they can help replace degenerated tendon tissue. Though promising, this therapy is not yet widely available. Several clinical trials are now ongoing. To find one, go to *Clinical Trials.gov.*

FROZEN SHOULDER

Frozen shoulder (or adhesive capsulitis), which usually occurs for unknown reasons, develops when the capsule surrounding the shoulder joint gets inflamed and then stiffens. A dull ache in the shoulder can come and go, slowly worsening to a ferocious pain that may awaken you during sleep or hurt even when your arm is at your side.

In the past, doctors recommended physical therapy to "thaw out" the joint and restore range of motion. But the physical therapy typically aggravated the condition—and it often did not improve for more than a year.

Recent thinking: With a two-part approach—a cortisone injection given early on into the joint and gentle exercises—sufferers can get pain relief and restore their range of motion within a matter of weeks to months.

Surgery is rarely needed if frozen shoulder is promptly diagnosed and treated at this stage. Cortisone injections are usually not helpful when frozen shoulder has progressed to se-

vere stiffness, but physical therapy may help restore mobility.

After receiving a cortisone injection, the following exercises should be performed on the recovering shoulder three times a day. *Gently hold each for five seconds and do 10 reps of each exercise…*

•**Overhead stretch.**

What to do: Lie on your back with your arms at your sides. Lift your arm straight up in the air and over your head. Grab your elbow with your other arm and gently press toward your head.

•**Cross-body reach.**

What to do: Stand and lift your arm to the side until it's a bit below shoulder height, then bring it to the front and across your body. As it passes the front of your body, grab the elbow with your other arm and exert gentle pressure to stretch the shoulder.

•**Towel stretch.**

What to do: Drape a towel over the unaffected shoulder, and grab it with your hand behind your back. Gently pull the towel upward with your other hand to stretch the affected shoulder and upper arm.

Play a Tune for Better Sleep!

Playing a woodwind instrument (clarinet, flute or saxophone) for at least a half hour every day lowered risk for sleep apnea by 18%, a recent study of 129 adults found.

Possible reason: Better muscle tone in the upper airways prevents them from collapsing during sleep and causing the frequent pauses in breathing that occur with sleep apnea. Don't play an instrument? Singing could help, too.

Silas Daniel Raj, MD, researcher, Sree Balaji Medical College & Hospital, Tamil Nadu, India.

Torn Meniscus? Common Surgery for Knee Pain Works No Better Than Fake Surgery

Kenneth Fine, MD, orthopedic surgeon, The Orthopaedic Center, Rockville, Maryland, and assistant clinical professor of orthopedics, George Washington University School of Medicine and Health Sciences, Washington, DC. TheOrthoCenterMD.com

Your knee is killing you and the pain won't quit, so you consult an orthopedist. He says that you've torn your meniscus, one of two C-shaped pieces of cartilage in the knee that serve as shock absorbers and help lubricate the joint. Then he recommends arthroscopic surgery to repair or trim back the tear, assuring you that it's a very common and minimally invasive procedure.

Do you say OK to the operation? Hold your horses! Even though this surgery is the most frequently performed orthopedic procedure in the US, there's growing evidence that in many cases—or even in most cases—it simply doesn't help. In fact, according to a recent study, the procedure works no better than fake surgery! *Here's what your knees need you to know....*

REAL DEAL VS. A SHAM

The common treatment for a torn meniscus is an arthroscopic partial meniscectomy, in which a video camera and instruments are inserted through a few tiny incisions in the knee so the damaged portion of the meniscus can be trimmed away and smoothed out. It's the bread-and-butter procedure for many orthopedic surgeons, with 700,000 such procedures done each year in the US alone, at a cost of $4 billion. The study, which was done in Finland and published in *The New England Journal of Medicine*, included 146 men and women. All had knee pain consistent with a degenerative tear—the most common type, caused by the "wear and tear" of aging rather than a sudden injury—of the meniscus. All were prepped for surgery and given anesthesia (usually spinal but sometimes general). Once the tear was confirmed by arthroscopic examination, a nurse opened an envelope to reveal each

patient's random assignment to one of two study groups. The first group got the real operation...the second group got a sham procedure in which the surgeon simply pretended to operate.

With the real meniscectomy, the damaged and loose parts of the meniscus were removed with tiny instruments, including a shaver to smooth the torn edges. For the sham operation, the surgeon asked for the same surgical instruments, manipulated the knee as if he were operating, pushed the shaver (without the blade) on the outside of the knee and used suction. Either way, participants were kept in the operating room for the same amount of time. Afterward, all were given the same postoperative walking aids and instructions for a graduated exercise program to promote recovery. Neither the patients nor the doctors with whom they followed up after surgery knew which procedure—real or sham—each patient had undergone.

Startling results: When patients were evaluated a year later, both groups reported equal levels of improvement in their knees. There were no significant differences in pain scores for the two groups, and both groups were equally satisfied with the outcome of their procedures—in fact, 93% of the surgery group and 96% of the sham group said that, given the chance, they would have the same procedure again.

In other words, the fake surgery was just as effective as the real deal!

IS THE TEAR CAUSING THE PAIN...OR NOT?

So what the heck is going on? When a patient has knee pain, his doctor typically orders an MRI...and if the MRI shows that the meniscus is torn, the pain is generally assumed to be attributable to the tear. However, that assumption could be wrong.

Evidence: A study of nearly 1,000 randomly selected men and women ages 50 to 90 showed that one-third of them had meniscus tears. Tears were more common among the older people than the younger ones, which makes sense because these generally are considered wear-and-tear injuries that increase with age. What was startling was that the majority of tears (61%) were found in people who had no symptoms—no knee pain, no stiffness, no swelling. Furthermore, participants who had arthritis in the knee (as shown on x-rays) were more likely to have tears, even if they didn't have knee pain...and the worse the arthritis was in a given person, the higher the likelihood that that person had a meniscus tear.

What does this mean? In many cases, a torn meniscus could be an early sign of arthritis rather than the source of knee pain. It would be the arthritis—not the tear in the meniscus—causing the pain.

Arthritis of the knee is extraordinarily common, with more than 9 million men and women in the US having x-ray evidence of the disease and symptoms. Up until a few years ago, many people with arthritis of the knee had an operation to "clean out" the joint—until several studies showed that the operation is just not helpful. In fact, some studies suggested that arthritis progresses more rapidly in people who have had an arthroscopic meniscectomy.

In many cases, it's likely that the pain is from the arthritis and not the meniscus tear. A basic principle is that surgery is good for fixing mechanical problems but not for curing pain. People with knee pain can become frustrated, and they want to 'do something'—but often surgery is just not the answer.

WHAT HELPS WHEN SURGERY WON'T

For patients with knee pain and meniscus tears, especially the degenerative type, start conservatively. Interventions don't do anything directly to the meniscus, but they can help maintain the basic overall functioning of the knee. *Consider some or all of the following approaches...*

• **Temporary "activity modification"**—for instance, if you play a lot of tennis, you may need to cut back on your time and/or intensity until your knee feels better.

• **Ice packs applied for 20 minutes at a time,** several times a day.

• **Strengthening exercises for the quadriceps and hamstring muscles that help support the knee,** such as those recommended by the American Academy of Orthopaedic Surgeons (*www.aaos.org*).

• **Physical therapy** to further strengthen muscles and extend the range of motion.

• **Oral anti-inflammatory medications,** such as aspirin or ibuprofen, as needed.

• **A cortisone injection in the knee to reduce inflammation.**

• **Weight loss,** if appropriate.

WHEN IS AN OPERATION WARRANTED?

This is not to say that meniscus surgery is never justified. *An operation may well be the best bet for...*

• **Patients with degenerative tears that have resulted in a small piece of cartilage getting curled up under itself or a flap of cartilage literally getting stuck in the joint.** An MRI sometimes can reveal such a problem, but often the doctor must make a clinical judgment as to its likelihood.

• **Patients who have acute tears (rather than degenerative tears) of the meniscus—** the type typically associated with sports injuries or other trauma. For one thing, acute tears sometimes can be repaired effectively with sutures instead of being trimmed. For another thing, addressing such injuries helps keep the rough torn edge of the meniscus from damaging the joint surface...and this is particularly important in younger people, who generally have firmer cartilage than older people do. In contrast, degenerative tears tend to be smoother and the cartilage softer, so they usually do no additional harm to the knee.

Bottom line: If you've been told that you need surgery for a torn meniscus, ask your doctor about the findings in this article...and if he doesn't make a clear case that your meniscus damage warrants surgery, get a second opinion before deciding whether to have the operation. You can get a referral from the American Academy of Orthopaedic Surgeons. After all, there's no point in putting yourself through the expense, inconvenience and risks that go along with any surgery if your knee is likely to improve just as much with some smart noninvasive therapies...plus time and patience.

The Buzz About Positional Therapy for Sleep Apnea

Lawrence J. Epstein, MD, program director of the Sleep Medicine Fellowship Program and associate physician, division of sleep and circadian disorders, departments of medicine and neurology at Brigham and Women's Hospital, and instructor in medicine at Harvard Medical School, all in Boston. Dr. Epstein also is past president of the American Academy of Sleep Medicine.

It happened again—a night's sleep was wrecked by the gasping for air, snoring and snorting caused by obstructive sleep apnea (OSA). The symptoms strike whenever you roll over onto your back, and even though you know a CPAP machine would fix the problem, you just can't get yourself to use one. You might even have a machine gathering dust in a corner of your bedroom.

No worries. If lying on your back really is what sets off your OSA, there is, in fact, a new way to avoid symptoms and get some shut-eye.

DON'T LET SLEEP APNEA GET YOU FLAT ON YOUR BACK

Half of people with OSA generally have symptoms only when they are sleeping on their backs. This is called positional OSA. Until recently, CPAP was the main and doctor-preferred treatment for positional OSA even though simply not sleeping on your back prevents symptoms, too. Studies have shown that, although not quite as effective as CPAP, positional therapy—which offers a variety of techniques to keep a sleeper off his or her back—is adequate to control OSA symptoms in people who won't or can't use a CPAP machine.

Until now, positional therapy has been pretty basic, involving use of low-tech objects such as tennis balls, body pillows or foam belts that discourage or prevent a person from rolling onto his back during sleep. Now, a new approach, called vibro-tactile positional therapy, uses vibration to prevent a person from sleeping on his back. And the device, called Night Shift, does not restrict movement like the older options do.

NO LOST SLEEP

Night Shift is a relatively thin neck collar with a sensor that vibrates when you roll onto your back. The intensity of the vibration increases until you change your sleep position.

Surprisingly, this vibrating gadget will not disrupt sleep and keep you up as much as your OSA will, says Lawrence J. Epstein, MD, an expert in sleep medicine and positional therapy from Harvard Medical School and past president of the American Academy of Sleep Medicine. Although you might be briefly roused to roll over, you usually won't completely awaken, he said. You simply will shift position and fall right back into deeper sleep.

The device also electronically monitors how often you roll onto your back, how long you stay in that position before shifting and how much you snore or have breathing problems during sleep, explained Dr. Epstein. "This information can be downloaded onto a computer and sent to your doctor to determine how effective the device is for you," he said.

According to a small published study sponsored by Advanced Brain Monitoring, Inc. (the makers of Night Shift) and conducted by the inventors of the device, Night Shift reduced sleep apnea by more than half in 83% of the study participants who used the device nightly for four weeks. This had a greatly improved effect on snoring, daytime depression and sleepiness and, most importantly, getting enough oxygen during sleep. At some point though, a larger, independent study will need to confirm Night Shift's effectiveness and also compare it to CPAP. But the bottom line is that using any technique that will help prevent OSA is better than nothing. OSA is a risk factor for cardiovascular problems, such as irregular heartbeat, high blood pressure and heart attack, and eye problems, such as glaucoma—so it is vital to do what you can to prevent it.

HOW TO GET THE DEVICE

Night Shift is available by prescription only, so if you want to try it, speak with your doctor. Dr. Epstein advised that it may be worth your while to see a board-certified sleep specialist rather than your primary care physician to get a prescription for the device. Unlike a primary care doctor, a sleep specialist (a physician with training and board certification in sleep medicine) can ensure that positional therapy is right for you. Such a doctor will also best use the product's technology to closely monitor your response to treatment.

Although Night Shift is not yet widely covered by insurance, at $349, it's about one-third of the price of a CPAP machine.

Drug-Free Magnet Therapy for Tough-to-Treat Depression

Noah Philip, MD, staff psychiatrist, Butler Hospital, and assistant professor of psychiatry and human behavior, Alpert Medical School of Brown University, both in Providence. Dr. Philip holds a special certificate in TMS from the International Society of ECT and Neurostimulation.

People with depression really do suffer… and for those who have what's called treatment-resistant major depression, psychotherapy and antidepressant medication just don't help.

The good news: Many such patients can be helped by transcranial magnetic stimulation (TMS), a noninvasive drug-free approach that used to be considered way-out-there experimental but is now finding its place in the mainstream.

A recent study from Brown University showed very encouraging results, given that it measured the success of TMS in the real world rather than in the rarified atmosphere of a research setting. The researchers followed 307 depression patients who were being treated with TMS at 42 different US-based medical practices. Though other therapies had failed for all of these patients, after receiving TMS, 58% experienced significant relief and 37% saw their depression go into remission.

"TICKLING" THE BRAIN

TMS is not the same as electroconvulsive ("shock") therapy—TMS uses electricity in a much gentler form. With TMS, electricity is transferred to the brain through an electro-

magnet to stimulate or "tickle" the prefrontal cortex, the part of the brain that allows us to think, plan, reason, hope and dream. The magnetic field lets the electrical current penetrate the skull and provide a "jump-start" for underactive mood-regulating brain circuitry.

Noah Philip, MD, an assistant professor of psychiatry and human behavior at the Alpert Medical School of Brown University, has been researching treatment-resistant depression for many years, including TMS. He said, "With TMS, we take a magnet that's roughly the same strength as those used in MRI scanners, though smaller, and we use it to deliver a series of rapid pulses of magnetic energy over parts of the brain that are involved in depression. We don't yet know exactly how it works, but we think that it changes the activity of individual neurons in the brain and makes them fire properly, alleviating the symptoms of depression."

WHAT TO EXPECT DURING TMS TREATMENT

Typically, TMS treatments take place in a doctor's office on an outpatient basis and last about 40 minutes each. Patients visit five days a week for six weeks, after which they usually need only a handful of follow-up visits. No anesthesia or sedation is required. While the patient sits in a reclining chair, a magnetic coil positioned on the left forehead delivers a very rapid series of electromagnetic pulses. Generally the pulses are delivered for four seconds, then there is a rest period of 26 seconds…then that sequence is repeated several dozen times.

Dr. Philip likened the sensation to "having a woodpecker tapping on your forehead"—a sensation that results from the nerves in the face being stimulated—so it's not exactly pleasant, but it doesn't really hurt. Some patients experience a twitching sensation of the scalp and/or brief headaches during the treatment, but otherwise there are no significant side effects. This is a distinct advantage over antidepressant medications, which can cause lowered libido, weight gain, headache, fatigue, anxiety and zombielike moods. Importantly, TMS does not cause memory problems the way electroconvulsive therapy does. Patients

16

can resume their normal activities immediately after the end of each session. There are no long-term safety concerns associated with being exposed to the electromagnetic energy, Dr. Philip said.

Who can be helped: TMS may be recommended for people with major depression who have tried one or more types of antidepressant medication without success. TMS is not appropriate for patients with seizure disorders because theoretically, with any stimulation of the brain, there is a risk of triggering a seizure (although Dr. Philip pointed out that in clinical trials involving more than 10,000 TMS treatments, no seizures were reported). TMS also should not be used by people with metal implants in or near their heads, such as aneurysm clips, cochlear implants or stents for hydrocephalus. Dental fillings and other metal orthodontic work do not interfere with TMS. Patients with cardiac pacemakers or implantable cardioverter defibrillators who are interested in TMS must discuss the treatment with their doctors first, Dr. Philip said, because the various devices differ in whether they can tolerate TMS.

Researchers do not yet know how long TMS's benefits typically last. As with psychotherapy and antidepressant drugs, some patients do relapse after TMS. However, when this occurs, another round of TMS treatment can be used. Dr. Philip said, "For people who respond to a first round of TMS, the odds of responding to a subsequent round are as high as 80%."

Currently there is one FDA-approved device for TMS on the market, and it is in use at several hundred physician-run centers across the US. The treatment should be provided by a TMS-trained physician. Your doctor or psychiatrist can provide a referral, or you can check the device manufacturer's website at *www. NeuroStarTMS.com.*

The cost of a six-week course of treatment varies depending on the location and the provider. Because TMS is FDA-approved and is included in the American Psychiatric Association's Practice Guideline for the Treatment of Patients With Major Depressive Disorder, many major insurance companies are now covering the treatment—so check with your health insurer.

The Secrets of People Who Never Get Sick

Gene Stone, a health journalist based in New York City who, in the process of writing about health, has undergone dozens of treatments, from hypnotherapy to Rolfing. He interviewed more than 100 healthy people for his latest book, *The Secrets of People Who Never Get Sick.* SecretsOfPeople.com

W hy is it that some people hardly ever get sick? I wanted to learn their secrets. *Some of these secrets, I discovered, are a bit unusual, but they have a basis in scientific fact...*

BREWER'S YEAST

Barbara Pritzkat, age 84, hasn't had a cold in decades. In 1983, at age 56, she started her second career as an archaeologist. She's still surveying archaeological sites, most recently in the Syrian Desert, where temperatures can reach 110°F. She credits her good health to brewer's yeast, which she takes in powder form dissolved in water every morning. She first learned about the health benefits of brewer's yeast in the 1940s when she attended a lecture by Adelle Davis, a pioneering nutritionist.

The science: Most commercially available brewer's yeast is extracted from the yeast that is used to ferment beer or wine. A single tablespoon contains the recommended daily allowance for most of the B vitamins, including folate.

Folate is one of the most important B vitamins because it breaks down and eliminates homocysteine, an amino acid, from the blood. Reducing homocysteine has been linked to a reduction in risk for stroke and heart disease. Folate also is thought to reduce the risk for a variety of cancers, including colon cancer.

Other B vitamins are needed for the maintenance of blood cells, nerves and the immune system. Brewer's yeast also contains a variety of minerals, including chromium, a trace mineral that reduces blood sugar and improves glucose tolerance. In addition, a single two-ounce serving provides eight grams of protein, more than the amount in a large egg.

What to do: Take one to two tablespoons of brewer's yeast daily. You can dissolve it in water or sprinkle it on your cereal or yogurt. Some people may suffer adverse gastrointestinal reactions at first. Start by taking a small amount and increase it gradually.

Any brand should be fine—even buying from bulk bins. But look for a kind that's debittered—the taste is more palatable.

COLD SHOWERS

They're not very pleasant, but your shivering body may thank you.

Nate Halsey, age 38, got hooked on cold-water hydrotherapy a decade ago, when one of his friends explained that cold showers were the reason that he never got sick. Nate, who had been getting sick fairly often, gave it a try—and hated it. He still hates it, but he likes the energy boost. He also appreciates that he never gets sick anymore.

The science: Researchers have found that cold-water submersion increases levels of disease-fighting white blood cells. In one study, scientists found that people who took cold showers daily for six months had fewer colds than those in a control group. In another study, year-round swimmers in Berlin, who took regular dips in freezing-cold water in the winter, suffered half as many chest infections as other people.

Exposure to cold water also may increase glutathione, one of the body's main antioxidants—the study of Berlin swimmers found that they had elevated levels of glutathione.

What to do: Ease into it. Turn on the cold water for 30 seconds or so. With the shower running, stick your head in to wet your hair. Turn off the water, shampoo your hair, then turn the water back on to rinse off the lather and get your skin wet. Turn off the water again, soap your body, then turn the water back on to rinse off. The entire event should take about five minutes.

Editor's note: Recent research from Thrombosis Research Institute in London has found that cold water stimulates immune cell production and a one-minute cold shower (amid a nice hot shower) is enough to boost immunity.

Caution: If you have a heart condition, Raynaud's disease or blood pressure issues, talk to your doctor first.

GARLIC

Even people who do their best to take care of themselves aren't immune to colds and flu. That was the experience of Susan Brown, age 51, a shiatsu massage therapist and former owner of a health-food store. She got the flu year after year—until her boyfriend recommended garlic.

Now she cooks with garlic every day, adding it to every dinner, which often consists primarily of vegetables and some kind of starch, such as rice or pasta. She also squeezes raw garlic on top of the dish. If she feels like she's coming down with a cold, she eats garlic three times a day, and within 24 hours, she's fine. She hasn't gotten the flu since she started her garlic regimen more than six years ago.

The science: Garlic has antibacterial and antiviral properties. Researchers at the University of Western Australia found that people who began using garlic were able to reduce their sick days by more than 50%.

Some of the active ingredients in garlic inhibit the ability of platelets to form clots in the arteries—important for preventing heart disease and stroke. People who eat garlic regularly can have drops in blood pressure of about 10 mm Hg (millimeters of mercury).

What to do: Chew a clove of garlic whenever you feel a cold coming on or you want to give your health a quick boost. It's best consumed raw, as cooking may destroy some of its health benefits. Most scientific studies are done with garlic supplements. However, some experts believe that the process of making the supplements destroys some of the health benefits.

Caution: If you're on a blood thinner or have a bleeding disorder, such as hemophilia, talk to your doctor before consuming large amounts of garlic.

PROBIOTICS

Tony Japour, MD, age 51, is a molecular virologist and pharmaceutical researcher. His impressive credentials didn't keep him healthy. He would get a nasty cold every year. The colds stopped six years ago when he started consuming a yogurt drink that contains live bacterial cultures.

The science: Many of the bacteria that live in the digestive tract have beneficial effects. Known as probiotics, these organisms have been shown to relieve many gastrointestinal conditions and to boost the body's immunity, reduce blood pressure and decrease cholesterol.

Probiotics that live in the intestine make it harder for disease-causing germs to take up residence. People who have low levels of probiotics—after taking antibiotics, for example—get infections more often than those with healthy probiotic levels.

How to do it: Eat one or more servings of probiotic-rich foods daily. These include yogurt with live cultures, fermented soybean pastes (such as miso or tempeh), sauerkraut, probiotic-fortified soy milk and fermented cheeses, such as cottage cheese.

If you're not eating probiotic-rich foods, you can take a supplement. Look for one that has a blend of probiotic organisms, such as Lactobacillus (L.) acidophilus, L. rhamnosus and/or L. bulgaricus, and follow directions on the label.

PH BALANCE

Until about eight years ago, Thomas Appell, age 56, got a cold or the flu along with a sore throat at least two or three times a year. One of his healthier friends explained his own secret—no sugar, no meat and a lot of vegetables. Appell followed the diet and found that he stopped getting sick. He investigated why the diet was working and discovered that the foods he was eating were predominantly alkaline. The traditional American diet is highly acidic. It's possible that diseases thrive when the body's pH—a measure of acidity/alkalinity—is out of balance.

The science: Proponents of the pH theory of health argue that our shift away from a plant-based, low-protein diet, which naturally keeps the body's pH at "neutral" levels, created epidemic levels of disease.

Several recent books, including one from medical anthropologist and certified nutritionist Susan E. Brown, PhD, have linked disease to metabolic acidosis, which can occur when the kidneys don't process acids fast enough.

What to do: Before you can achieve an optimal pH, you have to know your baseline. You can buy pH test-strip kits at pharmacies and health-food stores. Basically, you hold a strip in your urine stream, then look at the color. Most experts recommend testing the first urine of the morning. A pH chart that comes with the kit explains the reading.

Most people will find that they're slightly acidic. To balance your pH, you will want to eat highly alkaline foods. These include most vegetables, legumes and olive oil. You also want to avoid foods that make your body more acidic, such as meats and processed foods. Thomas routinely checks his urine pH after a meal to see the food's effect on his balance.

Even critics of the pH balance theory agree that eating more vegetables and fewer processed foods is important for good health.

Fight Colds the Way Performers Do

Len Horovitz, MD, an internist, a pulmonary specialist and director of Carnegie Medical PC, a private practice in New York City. *New York Magazine* has included him among "The Best Doctors in New York" for both pulmonary and internal medicine. He is a contributor to the medical anthology *The Singer's Guide to Complete Health.*

When you catch a cold, the sneezing, runny nose, sore throat and coughing will most likely make you feel miserable for a week or so, yet you probably manage to go about your business.

But what if you were an opera singer or a Broadway actor and started sniffling a few days before opening night? Or a politician or a preacher? For these so-called "voice professionals" (individuals whose jobs require the use of their voices), a cold wreaks havoc on their ability to work. They can take cortisone (an anti-inflammatory steroid) to quickly relieve laryngitis, but congestion and other symptoms don't give up so easily.

As it turns out, there are a number of effective, unique therapies that voice pros use to prevent and treat colds and related illnesses...

COLDS

The average American catches two to four colds a year. Avoiding the common cold involves well-known precautions such as getting enough rest, drinking plenty of fluids, eating a nutritious diet and frequent hand-washing. But these don't always work.

For voice pros, if a cold or related illness does develop, they must deal with it before it gets bad enough to affect their ability to work. Their secrets...

•**Slippery elm tea.** Derived from the inner bark of the slippery elm tree, this traditional remedy eases coughs and sore throat pain. The bark contains mucilage, a substance that becomes slick and gel-like when mixed with water. It's a highly effective remedy for coating and soothing the throat.

To make this tea: Pour two cups of boiling water over about two tablespoons of powdered bark. Steep for five minutes and drink. Do this several times a day.

Or try slippery elm lozenges.

•**Lots of black pepper.** It's an expectorant that quickly thins mucus to reduce congestion. Add generous amounts to your meals whenever possible until you've gotten over your stuffy nose.

•**Fruit smoothies.** These tasty drinks will replenish lost fluids, and the antioxidants may even help you recover from a cold more quickly.

What to do: Once or twice a day, blend fruits—such as pineapple, blueberries and/or bananas—with a cup or two of fruit juice and some ice. Do not add anything else—the key is to get a potent shot of antioxidants and a

lot of liquid. (If you have diabetes, be sure to check with your doctor before using this remedy, since fruit contains high amounts of natural sugar.)

•**Zinc.** Used within 24 hours after symptoms start, zinc lozenges can shorten the duration of a cold by at least a day. Use the lozenges until the cold is gone, but don't take more than four lozenges a day.

•**Vitamin C.** Throughout cold season, take 500 mg of vitamin C twice a day to prevent colds...or 1,000 mg twice a day to recover from a cold more quickly. (If you get diarrhea from this dose, reduce the amount you take accordingly.)

LARYNGITIS

Most colds clear up in a week or so, but they're sometimes followed by laryngitis, inflammation of the larynx (voice box) that can last for several weeks.

In addition to resting your voice as much as possible, try this...

•**Steam with eucalyptus oil.** Few remedies are better than steam and eucalyptus, a powerful decongestant, for quick relief of laryngitis.

What to do: After boiling a couple of cups of water in a saucepan, turn off the heat and add a few drops of eucalyptus oil (available at health-food stores). Lean over the pan with a towel draped over your head to trap the steam. Being careful not to burn yourself, breathe the steam for a few minutes, two to three times a day.

SORE THROAT

A sore throat is usually due to a viral infection. If the pain is not severe—and the soreness starts to go away within a few days—you probably won't need medical treatment. If the pain doesn't go away, or it seems to be getting worse, see your doctor to check for strep throat.

For a simple sore throat...

•**Gargle.** Use a salt–baking soda solution. The salt draws fluids from the tissues and reduces swelling and pain. Baking soda makes the gargle more soothing.

What to do: Add about one-half teaspoon each of salt and baking soda to one cup of warm water...and gargle for 30 to 60 seconds.

Important: Do not gargle with commercial antiseptic mouthwash. Even though it temporarily reduces bacteria in the mouth, it may damage mucous membranes in the throat and increase the risk for infection.

A SURPRISING CAUSE OF HOARSENESS

If you're hoarse, but it's not due to a cold or overuse of your voice (as is often the case with singers, politicians, preachers and sports fans), there may be another cause—and it's often overlooked.

Laryngopharyngeal reflux (LPR) is a condition in which stomach acid backs up into the larynx or throat (pharynx). It's similar to what happens with heartburn—but without the typical "burn" in the chest. *What to do...*

• **Follow heartburn-prevention strategies.** The same steps that you follow to prevent heartburn—eating smaller meals...avoiding greasy, fatty foods...not eating within a few hours of going to bed...and raising the head of the bed a few inches—will also help prevent LPR.

• **Neutralize stomach acid.** Alginate is a compound that neutralizes acid and helps prevent it from surging out of the stomach. It is an active ingredient in heartburn products such as Gaviscon.

• **Try DGL.** Taken in pill or powder form before meals when you're feeling hoarse, deglycyrrhizinated licorice (DGL) helps prevent stomach acid from damaging the larynx. Drugs such as Prilosec have a similar effect, but they increase osteoporosis risk. DGL is a safer remedy.

Lasers That Relieve Pain, Lasers That Heal

Mark A. Stengler, NMD, is a naturopathic medical doctor and leading authority on the practice of alternative and integrated medicine. Dr. Stengler is author of the *Bottom Line Natural Healing* newsletter, author of *The Natural Physician's Healing Therapies* (Bottom Line Books). MarkStengler.com

Here's one kind of treatment that I'll bet your mainstream doctor doesn't recommend to you—cold laser therapy. I have in the past recommended this type of laser treatment for fat reduction. But cold laser therapy can do so much more than that.

Cold laser therapy, so called because it is unlike older types of lasers that use very hot, high-energy beams of light, also is known as low-level laser treatment (LLLT). I use LLLT in my clinic to relieve many types of musculoskeletal pain, including arthritis and strained or inflamed muscles, joints, tendons and ligaments. Because LLLT reduces inflammation and improves circulation, I also use it to treat conditions such as sinusitis...lymphedema (swelling due to a buildup of lymph fluid in an arm or a leg, which is particularly common after a mastectomy)...and tinnitus (a condition characterized by ringing in the ears). LLLT also has been shown to speed up wound healing and improve the symptoms of carpal tunnel syndrome. If you have any of these conditions, I urge you to look into LLLT.

HOW IT WORKS

One of the things that I really like about LLLT is that it is a nontoxic treatment with virtually no side effects. LLLT of one type or another has been in use for about 30 years, but the technology has become more effective and has increased in popularity in recent years. In LLLT, laser light passes harmlessly into the body's tissues without heating them. LLLT devices deliver energy units called photons to damaged cells. This stimulates and increases the cells' metabolic activity and, in essence, brings them back to health.

LLLT uses different wavelengths to penetrate to varying depths—from just below the skin's surface to four to five inches deep. Depending on the area being treated, the therapy may employ one or more wavelengths during a treatment session. The laser in my clinic, like many others now in use, enables me to vary the frequency of wavelengths.

Once these photons reach their target depth, they produce a variety of effects that help reduce pain and accelerate healing by…

•**Stimulating the molecules that cells burn for energy.** This increases general cell health and enhances the cellular repair process. In particular, photons appear to increase the production of cells that promote tissue regeneration and wound healing.

•**Reducing inflammation** by inhibiting the body's production of inflammatory substances.

•**Improving blood vessel dilation,** which increases blood flow to the treated area.

•**Inhibiting the pain-signaling activity of nerve cells.**

•**Increasing production of serotonin,** the neurotransmitter associated with well-being.

•**Enhancing immune activity in the area being treated.**

Numerous studies have demonstrated LLLT's effectiveness. One 2009 study published in *The Lancet* was an analysis of 16 randomized controlled studies of LLLT for neck pain. The researchers concluded that patients were about 70% more likely to experience reduced pain following LLLT, compared with those given a placebo treatment. Similarly, a 2008 study published in *American Journal of Sports Medicine* found that recreational athletes with chronic Achilles tendinopathy who received LLLT combined with therapeutic exercises had faster recovery times. The laser group recovered after four weeks of treatment, compared with 12 weeks for the control group, which received no laser therapy.

When I use LLLT, I usually pass the laser over the affected area for five to 10 minutes per treatment. I often administer one to two treatments per week until symptoms resolve. Many people notice at least some improvement in pain, soreness and stiffness after just one treatment, and 90% of my patients notice a significant reduction in pain within two to three treatments. Benefits can last from weeks to months depending on the individual and the problem being treated. If desired, LLLT also can be used in conjunction with other therapies, such as physical therapy, anti-inflammatory medications and acupuncture. Laser treatments for conditions such as sinusitis and tinnitus work similarly.

HOW LLLT COULD HELP YOU

For patients with acute or chronic pain, LLLT often is my first choice when it comes to treatment options.

Take Susan, for example. This 65-year-old patient had severe bursitis in her hip. She was in so much pain that she had to walk with a cane. Another doctor had recommended a cortisone injection to relieve the pain, but she wanted to see what other treatments were available. There was no question in my mind that LLLT would help her. After just one treatment, her symptoms improved dramatically. After three treatments, she felt so much better and had such increased mobility that she no longer needed the cane.

LLLT typically costs $50 to $75 per session. Some health insurance companies cover it. Many naturopathic doctors, physiotherapists, chiropractors and acupuncturists, as well as some holistic medical doctors, are trained in LLLT. When choosing a practitioner, ask whether he/she has attended formal seminars in this type of therapy.

People with cancerous tumors should not have this treatment because it may aggravate their condition. Lasers have not been tested on pregnant women.

Help for Old-Looking Hands

Prominent veins and tendons, thinning skin and brown spots (also known as "liver spots" or "sun spots") are very common as we age. Topical skin lighteners, such as over-the-counter Lumixyl, can be used at home. There are also many in-office treatments for brown spots and crepey skin, including chemical peels, microneedling and laser therapy.

Until recently, little could be done for the veiny hands that often betray our age. But the FDA has now approved Radiesse, a calcium-based volumizing filler that recontours hands and camouflages veins and tendons. Hyaluronic acid fillers have also been successfully used off-label for hand rejuvenation. The cost of these treatments is not covered by insurance.

Nelson Lee Novick, MD, clinical professor of dermatology, Icahn School of Medicine at Mount Sinai, New York City. DoctorNovick.com

Cool Way to Firm Up Sagging Skin

Neil S. Sadick, MD, clinical professor of dermatology, Weill Cornell Medical College, New York City, and a cosmetic dermatologist in private practice, Sadick Dermatology. SadickDermatology.com

Are you afraid of face-lifts? The pain, the anesthesia, not to mention the cost. And what if something goes wrong? Do you dream of something less drastic to try—preferably something that didn't involve knives or needles?

Here's that dream answered: the nonsurgical technology called Venus Freeze. The results aren't nearly as dramatic as those a face-lift might provide, but it is noninvasive and painless and costs significantly less than cosmetic surgery. The procedure uses radiofrequency energy and magnetic pulses to tighten sagging skin and smooth out wrinkles and cellulite on the face, neck, upper arms, belly, hips and/or thighs.

As one of the developers of Venus Freeze, I have been using the treatment in my practice for several years and have performed it on over 1,000 patients to date. A small number of people don't get the desired effect, but over 80% have significant improvement.

•**How it works.** The Venus Freeze apparatus consists of a boxy energy-generating unit plus a handheld applicator that looks similar to a computer mouse. The energy it emits

penetrates multiple layers of skin, uniformly heating the tissues to about 40°C (104°F). In response, the skin's fibers of collagen (protein-based connective tissue) immediately shorten and thicken, tightening the skin...and over the next several weeks, new collagen forms that provides additional support. Fat-cell volume also decreases, improving the appearance of cellulite. In addition, the treatment induces the release of growth factors needed for new blood vessel formations, thus promoting the flow of blood, nutrients and oxygen to the tissues.

Because Venus Freeze is fairly new, having been cleared by the FDA late in 2010, there isn't a lot of peer-reviewed research available yet (a fact that will no doubt give some people pause). However, one study recently published in *Journal of Dermatological Treatment* is promising—on a scale of one to 10, patients' average satisfaction level was eight and their average pain score was only 1.5.

In another study that I conducted, 31 patients (mostly middle-aged women) received 10 weekly or twice-weekly treatment sessions for facial wrinkles. None of the participants experienced pain, burns, skin damage or scarring. Three months later, when an independent dermatologist and a plastic surgeon analyzed before-and-after photos, 97% of patients received improved scores on a standard wrinkle scale.

There are no long-term safety risks with Venus Freeze (though people who have concerns about any possible risks that might be associated with other radiofrequency and/or electromagnetic devices—cell phones, microwave ovens, overhead power lines—may not feel comfortable with this new technology). *If you are interested in trying it, here's what you'll want to know...*

•**What it can and cannot do.** Venus Freeze is worth considering if you have fine facial wrinkles or jowls yet don't have a tremendous amount of sagging skin. But if your complexion is already showing considerable signs of aging, the treatment isn't for you.

As for using Venus Freeze elsewhere on the body, don't count on it to dramatically whittle your waistline, eliminate underarm jiggles or slenderize thighs—it's no substitute for good old-fashioned weight loss and toning exercises

23

or for liposuction. However, the technology can improve the appearance of mild-to-moderate cellulite and tighten loose skin in various areas. Venus Freeze is good for people with saggy skin on their upper arms or thighs and for women whose bellies remain stretched out after childbirth.

• **What to expect during treatment.** During this office procedure, the practitioner holds the applicator against the skin and moves it in continuous circular or sweeping motions. Each area takes about 10 minutes to treat. No anesthesia is needed—patients generally feel a slight sensation of warmth, if anything, and can return to normal activities immediately afterward. Side effects consist primarily of slight swelling and/or redness that fade within an hour. There is minimal risk for burns, Dr. Sadick said.

Venus Freeze is available in many areas of the country. To find a provider near you, check *www.VenusTreatments.com*. Before you settle on a practitioner, ask candidates the following questions…

• **"Who performs the treatment?"** You want a physician or physician assistant, not an aesthetician.

• **"How many patients have you treated with this technology?"**

Ideal answer: Opt for someone who has performed Venus Freeze on at least 25 patients.

• **"What does the treatment cost?"** This varies depending on your location and the area of the body being treated, but you can expect to pay several hundred dollars per session.

• **"How many sessions will I need?"** I usually recommend five to seven weekly treatments initially, with a follow-up session for maintenance every three to six months thereafter. Be skeptical if anyone promises to transform your skin in a single session…or tries to rope you into committing to a dozen or more sessions.

Mighty Mushrooms Combat Breast Cancer

Cynthia Bye, ND, naturopathic physician specializing in complementary cancer care at Journey to Wellness, her private practice in Vancouver, Washington. CynthiaBye.com

Cynthia Bye, ND, a naturopathic doctor based in Vancouver, Washington, often prescribes mushroom extracts for patients who want to be proactive in improving their immune function and reducing their cancer risk. And in fact, a growing body of research suggests that certain mushrooms are powerful weapons in the fight against breast cancer and other cancers. *For instance, various mushrooms…*

• **Contain chemicals (including conjugated linoleic acid) that act as aromatase inhibitors.** Aromatase is an enzyme in fat tissue that converts testosterone to estrogen. Since estrogen fuels many breast tumors, certain mushrooms combat breast cancer by suppressing aromatase activity.

• **Increase apoptosis, the natural programmed death of old, worn-out cells.** This acts as a check against the cells becoming cancerous (since cancer cells proliferate instead of undergoing apoptosis).

• **Stimulate the immune response through the action of beta glucans,** substances that support the production and/or function of various disease-fighting cells, including white blood cells, T-cells and natural killer cells.

Simply eating more mushrooms may be good for you—but for maximum therapeutic effects, consider mushroom extracts.

Reason: The beta glucans are in the mushrooms' cell walls, which you cannot digest. To get the beta glucans, Dr. Bye said, you need mushroom supplements prepared through a process called hot water extraction.

Dr. Bye recommended using mushroom extracts only under the guidance of a naturopathic doctor who is trained in their use, to assure that you receive a formulation specifically tailored to your needs. Mushrooms come in many different varieties—coriolus, crimini, maitake, portobello, reishi, shiitake, white button, etc.—and each has its own distinct health benefits. The extracts best suited to helping a healthy person stay healthy are not the same as those that might be prescribed for a person with compromised immunity…or for a woman at high risk for cancer…or for a woman with a history of breast cancer who wants to reduce the risk for recurrence. (See the following article for more on mushroom extracts.)

Referrals: American Association of Naturopathic Physicians (866-538-2267, *www.Naturopathic.org*).

Mushroom Extract May Hold Key to Pancreatic Cancer Cure

Daniel Sliva, PhD, senior investigator, Cancer Research Laboratory, Methodist Research Institute, Indiana University Health, Indianapolis. His study was published in *International Journal of Oncology.*

Michael Landon, Luciano Pavarotti, Sally Ride, Jack Benny, Patrick Swayze. Those are familiar names of people who have died from pancreatic cancer. You probably know someone who has succumbed to it as well, given that it is the fourth-leading cause of cancer-related deaths in the US.

Pancreatic cancer moves fast—many of its victims die within months of being diagnosed, and the five-year survival rate is dismal, not even reaching 5%. That's why any good news about pancreatic cancer is most welcome. So it's heartening to learn that a traditional Asian remedy made from mushrooms may hold the key to winning the battle against this dreaded disease, according to a new laboratory study.

MAGIC MUSHROOMS?

Poria cocos is a type of mushroom that grows on pine trees. Among practitioners of traditional Asian medicine, the mushroom has been used for many years as a sedative, diuretic and stomach settler. Recent studies suggested that bioactive compounds in mushrooms might protect against breast and skin cancer…so researchers set out to discover whether they also might hold promise against pancreatic cancer, for which there is no known cure.

For the new study, normal pancreatic cells and pancreatic cancer cells were laid out in culture trays in a laboratory, then treated with extracts from the Poria cocos mushroom to see how the cells would react.

Exciting: Within just one day, the mushroom extract inhibited several different mechanisms by which pancreatic cancer proliferates—so that the cancer cells acted less aggressively and didn't multiply as rapidly as they usually would. For instance, the mushroom extract seemed to silence one particular gene, MMP-7, that is overactive in pancreatic cancer cells. Importantly, the mushroom extract had minimal effect on the normal pancreatic cells.

Of course, these findings do not mean that pancreatic cancer patients can be cured by eating pine tree mushrooms. But scientists are already working on the next phase of research to determine exactly how the mushroom extract turns down the MMP-7 gene…and whether the extract has the same effects in real life as it does in the lab.

Cause for hope: The potent drugs morphine, penicillin and *paclitaxel* (Taxol, which is used to treat lung, breast and ovarian cancers) were derived from poppy plants, mold and Pacific yew tree bark, respectively. So it's not at all far-fetched that a mushroom might eventually prove to play a pivotal role in curing deadly pancreatic cancer.

2

Hidden Healthcare Dangers and Rip-Offs

Don't Let Your Doctor Get It Wrong

Fifteen years ago, my teenage son Lewis went to the hospital for an elective surgical procedure. After the operation, his doctors failed to notice that he was suffering from an undetected infection and blood loss from an ulcer caused by pain medication. They believed his symptoms were an indication of constipation from other pain medications he was taking. This mistake cost my son his life—he died four days after entering the hospital.

Now: I teach patients skills that can help them avoid a similar tragedy.

A "BLIND SPOT" IN MEDICINE

A groundbreaking new report from the prestigious Institute of Medicine (IOM) concluded that most Americans will experience at least one diagnostic error—that is, an inaccurate, missed or delayed diagnosis, as determined by later definitive testing—at some point in their lives.

The IOM report called diagnostic errors a "blind spot" in the delivery of quality health care. Each year, about one in 20 patients who seek outpatient care will suffer from a wrong or delayed diagnosis. According to autopsy studies, diagnostic mistakes contribute to about 10% of patient deaths. Unfortunately, diagnostic errors haven't gotten as much attention as treatment and surgical errors—for example, operating on the wrong body part—partially because the latter are easier and quicker to identify. Now patient-safety experts are taking steps to better understand why diagnostic errors occur. *Key reasons...*

•**Tests help—and hurt.** Patients may be given a staggering number of tests—X-rays, blood tests, biopsies and more. The process

Helen Haskell, MA, president of Mothers Against Medical Error, a nonprofit patient-safety organization, MAM Emomsonline.org. She serves on the board of directors of the National Patient Safety Foundation and is a board member of the Institute for Healthcare Improvement and the International Society for Rapid Response Systems. In 2015, she was named one of the top 50 patient-safety experts in the country by Becker's Hospital Review.

of ordering, conducting and conveying the results of a test, however, can be complex and poorly organized.

• **Poor communication.** Can you count on the internist to talk to the nurse? Will the radiologist convey all of the pertinent information to the surgeon? Don't count on it. Patients also play a role. They should tell their doctors about all the symptoms they're having and whether they're getting better or worse after starting a new treatment.

• **Snap judgments.** Doctors often develop a working diagnosis within the first few minutes of hearing the patient's reported symptoms. The danger is that doctors can develop a so-called anchoring bias that leads them to cling to their initial diagnosis and prevents them from fully considering new information or looking for other possibilities.

HOW TO MAKE SURE YOUR DOCTOR GETS IT RIGHT

Major medical groups, including the Society to Improve Diagnosis in Medicine, have identified a number of institutional factors—such as stronger teamwork—to reduce errors. But no one has more at stake in these situations than the patients themselves. *Four steps you can take to avoid a misdiagnosis…*

STEP 1: Organize your thoughts. Most of the time, doctors have only 15 minutes with each patient, so you need to make the most of your time together.

Plan ahead: Your medical history—including a description of symptoms and when the problem started—is the most important part of an exam. Describe the nature and context of your symptoms in as much detail as you can. When do you feel them? What makes them worse or better? Why are you worried? Keep it concise and on topic, but include your own thoughts so the doctor can address the issues that concern you.

My advice: If possible, before you see the doctor, use the Internet to investigate your symptoms and the likely causes. Your findings should not be used to challenge your doctor, but rather as a way to have a more informed conversation. If you don't have confidence in your own abilities to do research, take advantage of

a service like Expert HealthSearch (*ImproveDiagnosis.org/?page=ExpertHealthSearch*), a free service that puts you in touch with a medical librarian who can search the literature for you.

STEP 2: Don't be afraid to question test results. They are more prone to error than most people imagine. In one study, experts who reviewed biopsies of more than 6,000 cancer patients concluded that 86 had been given a wrong diagnosis. Samples can be too small or even contaminated…technicians can make mistakes…and there can be false-negatives or false-positives. Results can be misinterpreted, or even more often, they can go unreported to the patient.

My advice: If a test result seems to fly in the face of the symptoms you are experiencing, consider asking to repeat the test or have a second doctor review it. And never assume that no news is good news. Follow up to be sure that your test results have been received and reviewed and that you know what they are.

STEP 3: Ask about alternatives. Many common symptoms—such as fatigue, muscle aches and abdominal pain—are known as nonspecific symptoms. They can be caused by dozens of conditions.

My advice: To help understand your doctor's thinking, ask him/her this question: Could you please explain your differential diagnoses? This is a list of possible diagnoses ranked in order of likelihood. It's a thought process that helps a diagnostician avoid overlooking any likely possibilities. The most serious conditions on the list should be ruled out before settling on a less serious diagnosis, and the doctor should be looking for causes and not just treating symptoms.

What to ask: If there is any question about a diagnosis, patients can help assess the "fit" by asking three important questions: Does this diagnosis match all my symptoms? What else could it be? Could there be more than one thing going on?

STEP 4: Don't skip the second opinion. I cannot stress this enough. In the study of cancer patients cited earlier, Johns Hopkins University researchers found that one to two of every 100 who got a second opinion with definitive testing after a tumor biopsy had gotten a wrong diagnosis the first time.

My advice: It's not always possible to get a second opinion—sometimes in medicine you have to move fast. But if you can, a second (or even a third) opinion is smart when symptoms seem severe…if your doctor is recommending surgery…or if you are told that you have a rare or fatal condition. Check first, but usually insurance will pay for a second opinion. Outside of emergencies, most of the time a brief delay in treatment while you get a second opinion will not affect your outcome.

The Overdose Danger

Jack E. Fincham, PhD, RPh, a professor of pharmacy administration at Presbyterian College School of Pharmacy in Clinton, South Carolina. He is also a former panel member of the FDA Nonprescription Drugs Advisory Committee and currently serves on grant review panels for the Canadian Institutes of Health Research Drug Safety and Effectiveness Network.

When you get a new prescription, the first thing your doctor does (after choosing the drug) is decide on the dose.

What most people don't think about: Your doctor's dosing decision is crucial—getting even slightly more of a medication than you need can greatly increase your risk for side effects. Correct dosing, however, can lessen (or even eliminate) side effects.

Each year in the US, drug side effects are estimated to cause more than one million hospitalizations and more than 100,000 deaths. Yet many doctors reflexively prescribe "average" doses without checking recommendations for optimal dosing based on such factors as age, sex and body weight.

For example, a 100-pound woman might be given the same dose as a 200-pound man… and a 75-year-old may be given the same dose as a healthy college student. It's not hard to guess who is more likely to have preventable side effects. While many people know that taking a blood thinner in a dose that's too high can have devastating consequences, recent research is focusing on other drugs that can also have dangerous side effects.

Important new finding: With blood pressure drugs and diabetes medication, in particular, excessive doses can increase risk for dizzy spells, confusion, falls and even death—especially among adults age 70 and older, according to recent research in *JAMA Internal Medicine*.

DOSING DANGERS
Common drugs to watch out for…*

• **Blood pressure drugs.** About 25% of patients who take one or more of these medications stop using them within six months because of side effects, and up to half quit taking them within a year. The majority of people who take blood pressure drugs will initially suffer from dizziness, unsteadiness, falls or other side effects. Alert your physician if you experience any of these side effects. Even though the discomfort typically wanes over time, it can often be prevented altogether by starting with a lower dose of medication.

Beta-blockers, such as *metoprolol* (Lopressor) and *propranolol* (Inderal), are particularly dose-sensitive. So are alpha-blockers, such as *prazosin* (Minipress). Women who take these drugs tend to have a greater drop in blood pressure/heart rate than men, so they typically need a lower dose. The same may be true of patients who have both high blood pressure and lung disease, who often suffer shortness of breath when they take excessive doses. People who take multiple blood pressure medications are also more likely to have side effects.

My advice: Tell your doctor that you would like to start with one drug. Emphasize that you'd like to take the lowest possible dose—and that you're willing to be retested (or check your own blood pressure at home with an automated blood pressure monitor) to make sure that the treatment is working.

• **Diabetes medications.** The risks for diabetes complications—such as nerve damage, blindness, stroke and heart attack—are so great that doctors tend to treat it aggressively. But oral diabetes drugs given in high doses can easily cause blood sugar to fall too low.

*Never change a medication dose without consulting your doctor.

Example: Patients who take *glyburide* (Micronase) or *repaglinide* (Prandin) often develop hypoglycemia, excessively low blood sugar that can cause dizziness, confusion and other symptoms. Even if the initial dose was correct, physiological changes as you age and/or changes in your lifestyle could make that starting dose too potent. For example, suppose that you start exercising more and eating a healthier diet. You'll probably need a lower drug dose than you did before, but your doctor might not think (or know) to change the prescription.

My advice: Tell your doctor right away about any lifestyle changes that could affect your blood sugar levels, such as exercise frequency (or intensity), changes in meal timing, etc. Keep careful tabs on your blood sugar with home tests. If your blood sugar is consistently testing at the lower end of the recommended range (or below it), call your doctor and ask whether you should switch to a lower drug dose.

• **Painkillers.** Aspirin, *ibuprofen* (Motrin) and other nonsteroidal anti-inflammatory drugs (NSAIDs) are widely available and effective. But they're also dangerous at high doses. One study found that more than 70% of people who take these drugs daily on a regular basis suffer at least some damage to the small intestine. Like the blood thinner warfarin (Coumadin), they're a common cause of excessive bleeding.

My advice: Take the lowest possible dose… use painkillers as rarely as possible…and always take them with food. People assume that over-the-counter drugs are safe, but none of these medications are meant to be used long term (more than four weeks).

If you can, switch to one of the many brands of acetaminophen (such as Tylenol). It has about the same pain-relieving effects, but even with its increased risk for liver damage, acetaminophen (taken at the recommended dosage) is less likely than an NSAID to cause side effects.

• **Sedatives.** Valium and related drugs, known as benzodiazepines, are commonly prescribed sedatives in the US, but the standard doses can be much too high for women as well as older adults.

Medications such as *diazepam* (Valium), *triazolam* (Halcion) and *zolpidem* (Ambien) accumulate in fatty tissue. Since women have a higher percentage of body fat than men, the drug effects can linger, causing next-day drowsiness or a decline in alertness and concentration. In older adults, the drugs are metabolized (broken down) more slowly, causing unacceptably high levels to accumulate in the body.

My advice: Women who are given a prescription for one of these drugs should always ask if the dose is sex-specific. They can ask something like, "Do I need a lower dose because I'm a woman?"

Also, in my opinion, people age 65 or older should avoid these drugs altogether unless they have to take them for a serious problem, such as a seizure disorder. If your doctor says that you need a sedative, ask if you can use a shorter-acting drug such as lorazepam (Ativan)…if you can take it for a short period of time (less than a month)…or if you can get by with a lower dose.

Important: These drugs should never be combined with alcohol. The combination increases the sedative effects.

To learn more about a drug you're taking: Go to *Drugs.com*.

Is Your Doctor Scamming You with "Self-Referrals"?

Jean Mitchell, PhD, economist and professor of public policy, McCourt School of Public Policy, Georgetown University, Washington DC. She has written numerous articles on physician self-referral arrangements and other health-care economic topics.

Imagine: Your knee hurts. Your orthopedist says that he needs to do an MRI…and for your convenience, he has an MRI machine just down the hall. After checking your scan, the orthopedist recommends surgery, which can be done at an adjoining outpatient surgery center…after which you'll attend physical therapy, again conveniently located in the doctor's office complex.

Hassle-free, one-stop medical care for the patient? Or a money-making racket for the doctor?

Consider: If your doctor owns or leases the MRI machine used to examine your knee or if he owns part of the surgery center and/or physical therapy center, he is making money on every phase of your examination and treatment. He not only collects his professional fees for your office visit, but he also shares in any profits generated by the scan, the surgery or the physical therapy.

Those are huge monetary incentives.

Of course, it's quite possible that you really need the MRI, the operation and the physical therapy. But the doctor's financial involvement in so many of your health-care services creates a serious conflict of interest that makes it hard to know whether he is protecting your well-being or his own bottom line.

A TOOTHLESS LAW

The process described above is called self-referral, and in many circumstances, it's illegal. The federal government prohibits doctors from referring patients to facilities in which they have a financial interest. This regulation, known as the Ethics in Patient Referrals Act or the Stark Law (after the congressman who sponsored the bill), applies only to Medicare and Medicaid patients, but about half of the states have similar laws that apply to privately insured patients.

The loophole problem: The law is simply not enforced…and there are loopholes so big you can fit an MRI machine through them. The biggest loophole is the in-office ancillary services exception, which allows doctors to self-refer if the service is provided by them or by members of their practice in their office—which pretty much takes the teeth right out of the law.

Doctors have figured out other ways to circumvent the law, too. For example, a medical practice can enter into a contract with an independent imaging facility and agree to pay the facility a reduced, set fee for each service performed (a practice called payment per click). The referring doctor then bills the insurance company for the full-price service—and pockets the difference between what he collects from the insurance company and what he pays the imaging facility.

OVER-EVERYTHING

The biggest problems with self-referral involve three types of overutilization of health care…

Overtesting: Self-referral can lead to a lot of unwarranted tests, many of which carry risks. For instance, CT scans and X-rays involve radiation…the contrast materials used in some CT and MRI scans can cause kidney problems or allergic reactions…biopsies can be painful and can leave scars…and testing is highly stressful, particularly as anxious patients await the results.

Does ownership really affect doctors' decisions about the amount of testing to do? You bet it does. *Consider this evidence from recent studies…*

• **Doctors who owned imaging centers or leased imaging equipment referred their patients for imaging tests more than twice as often,** on average, as doctors in the same specialties but without this financial interest.

• **Patients of doctors who owned or leased MRI machines were 33% more likely to have normal MRIs than patients of doctors who didn't have MRI machines**—because owner-doctors were less selective in determining which patients really needed the test.

• **Male patients who had prostate biopsies** performed by doctors with an ownership interest in the pathology lab had 72% more specimens examined than patients of doctors without a financial interest—yet the patients of the lab-owning doctors were less likely to actually have cancer.

Overtreating: As if unwarranted tests weren't bad enough, self-referring doctors on average provide more unneeded treatments, too. Examples from recent studies…

• **Surgeons** who were partial or full owners of surgery centers performed at least twice as many of five studied procedures (such as knee arthroscopy and carpal tunnel surgery) as non-owner surgeons in the same specialties.

• **Prostate cancer patients being treated by urologists** who owned the equipment needed to perform intensity-modulated radiation therapy (IMRT) were nearly three times more likely to undergo this expensive treatment than men treated by urologists who did not own IMRT equipment.

•**Doctors who purchased IMRT equipment more than quadrupled their use of this treatment after acquiring the equipment, on average**—even though studies show that for low-risk disease (which accounts for the vast majority of prostate cancers), IMRT is no better than other treatments that cost about half as much. However, before these urologists purchased their IMRT equipment, they were no more likely than non-owner urologists to refer patients for IMRT.

Overcharging: Even when a test or procedure is necessary, the "convenience" of self-referral comes at a price. For instance, a recent study showed that for imaging tests, with the exception of X-rays, fees are higher, on average, when doctors self-refer patients rather than sending patients elsewhere for services. Even if you don't pay directly for those medical expenses, the excess costs still affect you—and everyone else—in the form of increased insurance premiums and copays.

How can consumers protect themselves in this era of self-referral? As patients, we don't have the clinical expertise to know whether we truly need a particular procedure, so we rely on our physicians to act as our agents. But when a physician is motivated by financial incentives, he may err on the side of recommending a test or procedure even if the patient is likely to have minimal or no benefit.

SELF-DEFENSE AGAINST SELF-REFERRAL

Until such time as the law is fixed and enforced, what can you do to protect your own health and wallet rather than the doctors' financial interests?

•**Ask your doctor directly whether he/she is self-referring.** When your doctor recommends a test or treatment, you can say point-blank, "Doctor, do you have any financial interest in this test or treatment?" If the answer is yes, inquire whether the results of the test will affect the treatment decision (if it won't, there's no reason to get the test)…and whether a particular treatment is the gold standard for your condition (if it isn't, the doctor should have a darn good explanation for why

he's recommending it). You can keep your eyes open for subtler clues, too.

•**Get a second opinion.** Consulting a second physician, especially before having an operation or starting a treatment program, is always a good idea. Just be sure that second doctor is not in the same practice as the first doctor—and again, ask this second doctor whether he's self-referring.

•**Feel free to go elsewhere for services.** You are under no obligation to limit yourself to the providers and facilities that your doctor recommends. Consider seeing a doctor who's on staff at a hospital associated with a university—these practitioners may be more likely to follow established guidelines on testing and treatment. Doctors on hospital staffs are frequently on salary, so although they may feel some indirect pressure from their institutions, they are less likely to be motivated by direct financial incentives.

Bottom line: If you have explored your options and decided that the convenience of a self-referral outweighs the downside, that's your right. Just don't let yourself be unwittingly herded into tests or treatments that do little more than create revenue for your doctor.

7 Ways to Make Outpatient Surgery Safer

David Sherer, MD, an anesthesiologist and former physician-director of risk management for a major HMO in the metropolitan Washington, DC, area. He is author, with Maryann Karinch, of *Dr. David Sherer's Hospital Survival Guide* and *The House of Black and White*, a memoir of growing up in a medical family. DrDavidSherer.com

E ver since Joan Rivers died after a routine surgical procedure at an outpatient center in Manhattan, people have been wondering if they're better off having surgery in a hospital.

The reality is that the vast majority of outpatient procedures go off without a hitch. But you can reduce your risk by getting involved before the procedure. Important steps…

CHECK YOUR PHYSICAL STATUS

Ask your doctor about your "physical status classification." The American Society of Anesthesiologists uses a numerical scale to assess a patient's surgical risks. Patients with higher physical status (PS) scores (four or five) because of health problems should have procedures done in hospitals because their risk for complications is higher.

Example: A patient who needs a knee replacement also might have poorly controlled diabetes, kidney insufficiency and nerve damage. His/her PS might be rated as four—too high to safely have a major procedure at an outpatient center.

In general, patients with PS scores of one through three—with one being generally healthy and three indicating that they have serious diseases that aren't life-threatening—are good candidates for outpatient procedures.

PICK YOUR SURGEON CAREFULLY

Don't assume that every surgeon in an outpatient center has the same experience—or the same credentials.

Suppose that you're planning to get Botox or Restylane injections. These are not as simple as most people think. For the best results—and the lowest risk for complications—you should have the procedure done by a physician who is board-certified in plastic and reconstructive surgery.

Caution: In many states, many procedures can be done by any physician who has undergone minimal training in these procedures, such as a weekend course or three-day seminar. These doctors might be board-certified in something but not necessarily in the field that concerns you.

Also important: The amount of experience. Studies have clearly shown that doctors who do a lot of procedures have better results, with fewer complications, than those who do them less often.

Example: If I were planning to have LASIK eye surgery, I wouldn't feel comfortable seeing a surgeon who had done the procedure 50 times. I would want someone whose total cases numbered in the hundreds or even thousands.

INSIST ON PAIN CONTROL

Most people assume that their surgeons will do everything possible to minimize postoperative pain. Not true. Some doctors are reluctant to order strong painkillers on an ongoing basis because they worry that the patient will become addicted. Or they mainly use narcotics (opioids, such as codeine and morphine) that dull pain but can cause unpleasant and sometimes dangerous side effects, including impaired breathing, constipation, itching, nausea and vomiting.

Poorly controlled pain is among the most serious postoperative complications. It impairs immunity and increases the risk for infection...slows healing times...and can increase the risk for blood clots when patients hurt too much to move normally.

My advice: Tell your surgeon that you're terrified of pain. Ask what he/she plans to use to relieve your pain—and emphasize that you would like to avoid narcotics if at all possible.

Also, ask about *bupivacaine* (Exparel), a nonnarcotic anesthetic that was recently approved by the FDA. The active ingredient is encapsulated in liposomal (fat-based) particles and slowly released over 72 hours. When injected into the surgical area, it relieves pain as effectively as narcotics with fewer side effects.

BEWARE OF SUPPLEMENTS

Tell your doctor about everything that you're taking. Surgeons and anesthesiologists routinely ask patients about medications that they're using. They don't always think to ask about supplements.

This is a dangerous oversight because many supplements—along with garden-variety over-the-counter medications such as aspirin—can interact with the drugs that are used during and after surgery.

Examples: Garlic supplements increase the risk for excessive bleeding, particularly when they're combined with aspirin. The herbs ephedra and kava can interfere with anesthetics.

Patients who are taking natural remedies—including vitamin E, echinacea, ginseng, valerian and St. John's wort—should ask their doctors if they need to quit taking them. You may need to stop two weeks or more before the procedure. Aspirin should be discontinued two to three days before.

PLAN FOR THE WORST

Even routine procedures sometimes go south. Most outpatient surgical centers are equipped with crash carts (used for cardiac emergencies) and other equipment and drugs for handling serious complications—but some don't have these on hand.

Ask the surgeon if a crash cart will be available. *Also ask...*

•**Is there dantrolene (Dantrium)?** It can reverse a rare but deadly complication from anesthesia known as malignant hyperthermia. The drug is always stocked in hospitals, but an outpatient center might not have it.

•**Is there succinylcholine (Anectine, Quelicin)?** It's a fast-acting paralytic agent that assists doctors in quickly intubating patients who can't breathe—one of the most dangerous complications of anesthesia. It has been reported that Joan Rivers might have lived if this drug had been available.

DON'T PUT UP WITH NAUSEA

It is estimated that 30% of all postsurgical patients will experience nausea, retching or vomiting. These are among the most common surgical complications.

My advice: Tell your anesthesiologist/surgeon if you've suffered from surgery-related nausea in the past. He/she can administer *granisetron* (Kytril) or *ondansetron* (Zofran), which helps prevent nausea in most patients.

GET MOVING

Try to get moving as soon as you can. Surgeons used to recommend lengthy bed rest for postsurgical patients. They now know that it's better to move around as soon as possible to prevent constipation, urinary retention and muscle weakness, among other common complications.

As soon as you're able, get up and walk (with your doctor's permission, of course). If you can't stand right away, at least move in bed. Stretch your legs. Move your arms. Roll over, sit up, etc. Any kind of physical movement increases blood flow and improves recovery times. It also improves the movement of your lungs, which can help prevent postsurgical pneumonia.

The Big Olive Oil Hoax

Janet Bond Brill, PhD, RDN, FAND, is a registered dietitian nutritionist, a fellow of the Academy of Nutrition and Dietetics and a nationally recognized nutrition, health and fitness expert who specializes in cardiovascular disease prevention. Based in Allentown, Pennsylvania, Dr. Bond is the author of *Blood Pressure DOWN and Prevent a Second Heart Attack*. DrJanet.com

Olive oil has long been among the top go-to items for a heart-healthy diet. But you need to be smart when shopping for this health food. There are now plenty of mislabeled olive oil products that have insufficient amounts of the ingredients that help keep your arteries clean...are cut with cheaper oils...contain chemical additives...and/or come from a country other than what's highlighted on the label. So, how do you know that the bottle of olive oil in your shopping cart is not some adulterated, inferior oil? To avoid being tricked by these deceptive practices, here's what to look for when shopping for olive oil...

•**Single country of origin.** An olive oil label may say that it is produced in a particular country when, in fact, it was only bottled there. For example, "Product of Italy" does not necessarily indicate that the olives are grown or pressed in Italy—only that it was bottled there. Look for the phrase "Produced and Bottled," which means that the oil is actually produced and bottled in the place of origin listed on the label.

For olive oil with the very highest levels of anti-inflammatory plant chemicals known as polyphenols, look for these olive varieties: Coratina and Moraiolo from Italy...Cornicabra and Picual from Spain...and Koroneiki from Greece.

•**Certification seals.** The following governing bodies guarantee that the oil has passed extensive quality checks, so look for a product that includes one of these seals to identify a trustworthy, authentic olive oil.

•**International Olive Council** (IOC)

•**North American Olive Oil Association** (NAOOA)

- **California Olive Oil Council** (COOC)

- **Denominazione d'Origine Protetta** (DOP)

- **Protected Designation of Origin** (PDO)

- **"Extra virgin."** This term is given by governing bodies (see above) to only the purest and best of olive oils. With extra virgin, the oil is "cold pressed," which means that it has been extracted mechanically from the olives without the use of excess heat or chemicals—processes that would damage the fragile polyphenols. Extra virgin also has the most natural olive flavor, antioxidants, vitamins, minerals and other heart-healthy components of the ripe olive fruit. In general, extra-virgin oils have up to 10 times higher polyphenol content levels than lower-grade oils.

- **A dark bottle or can.** The anti-inflammatory plant chemicals in olive oil are fragile and highly susceptible to deterioration by light, heat and air. To keep the heart-healthy ingredients stable, buy olive oil in dark bottles or cans.

- **Expiration date.** Unlike fine wines, olive oil does not age well, so the fresher, the better. The expiration or "best-by" date should be no more than 18 months from the date of purchase. If the harvest date is given, it should be less than one year ago. To ensure freshness and the greatest health benefits, you should use olive oil as soon as possible after the container is opened.

- **Price.** A good olive oil is time-consuming to produce, so a quality product will cost up to $35 for a 17-ounce bottle. But if you want an olive oil that will help keep your ticker beating strong, it's worth it! You can find such olive oils online at *OliveandGourmet.com* or high-end specialty food stores.

Going to the Hospital for Surgery? Vitamin D May Protect Your Mind

Study titled "Association between pre-hospital vitamin D status and hospital-acquired new-onset delirium" by researchers in the department of medicine, Harvard Medical School, and Brigham and Women's Hospital, both in Boston, published in *British Journal of Nutrition*.

It's terrible what hospitals can do to you. We all know someone who checked into the hospital with his or her mind completely intact, but then quickly (especially if there was surgery) became confused and disoriented in a most disturbing way.

It's called hospital-acquired delirium. And, yeah, it's scary.

Delirium in the hospital is more common—and more dangerous—than you may think. It's a severe condition that mostly affects older patients (although not only older patients) and is often missed by hospital staff, especially in emergency rooms. If it's not treated promptly, it can lead to longer hospital stays and poor health outcomes, including permanent cognitive problems and even a higher risk for mortality. It's more common if there's already some cognitive impairment, but research shows that between 3% and 29% of "low risk" patients without any existing cognitive problems succumb to delirium after a hospital stay. A combination of surgery, infection, social isolation, dehydration, poor nutrition and mind-affecting pharmaceuticals such as painkillers, sedatives and sleeping pills can bring it on…quickly.

You can't control all of these factors, especially in the heat of the moment during emergency treatment. But researchers have discovered a nutritional factor that may protect against hospital-induced delirium…vitamin D.

D IS FOR…NO DELIRIUM

Researchers examined records of about 4,500 men and women (average age 59) who were admitted to one of two large teaching hospitals in Boston from 1993 to 2006. They included patients who had been tested before their hospitalization for blood levels of vitamin D and excluded those who had a history of delirium or dementia. Of all the patients, 198 (4%) were ultimately diagnosed with hospital-acquired new-onset delirium.

Their vitamin D levels told a story. Even after adjusting for age, sex, race, other illnesses and reason for hospitalization (medical or surgical), low preadmission vitamin D status was strongly associated with risk for hospital-acquired delirium.

A NO-BRAINER APPROACH TO PROTECTING THE BRAIN

It's an observational study, which means it can't prove (or disprove) that a lack of vitamin D caused delirium, so it's possible that whatever caused delirium in these patients also made their vitamin D levels plummet. Nor does this study show that bringing vitamin D levels up to speed proactively prevents delirium. More studies will be needed to explore that hypothesis.

But it's a reasonable hypothesis, and there is good reason to believe that vitamin D may play a specific role in protecting the brain and the mind. The brain has vitamin D receptors throughout, and there is evidence that the active form of vitamin D may remove plaque, a hallmark of Alzheimer's, from brain cells, scientists have recently discovered. Research has shown that low blood levels of vitamin D are linked with dementia, Alzheimer's disease and depression.

In a way, though, the exact question is beside the point. Medicine is about balancing benefit and harm, and in this case, if you're vitamin D–deficient, there's no harm, and potentially much benefit, in bringing your body's vitamin D level up to normal! According to the National Institutes of Health, 77% of Americans are deficient in vitamin D, with blood levels under 30 ng/mL, and 6% have levels under 10 ng/mL. Even if you don't know your level, taking a daily supplement that contains up to 2,000 IU or 3,000 IU is considered safe.

An even better idea: Get a blood test. It's simple, quick, and inexpensive. If your level is low, your health-care provider may prescribe a higher dosage for a while or even recommend vitamin D injections to get your level up to normal quickly.

If you are going into the hospital or know someone who is, the idea of getting tested for vitamin D beforehand…and reaching a normal level with a supplement if need be…is a no brainer. It may prevent a scary form of delirium that can take hold in the hospital and lead to a downward health spiral. Even if it doesn't, it's a healthy thing to do.

MORE WAYS TO PREVENT HOSPITAL DELIRIUM

Whether it's you or a loved one, make sure that items such as eyeglasses or hearing aids are readily available, books and other familiar objects are nearby, and that the patient walks around if possible, stays hydrated, and gets as much sleep as possible in the sleep-depriving hospital environment. Regular visits from friends and family are key, since being (and feeling) isolated can lead to loneliness and fear that in turn can be a factor in delirium. Monitor medications carefully, especially pain and sleep drugs, which can contribute to confusion and push a patient toward delirium. If you're caring for a loved one who does become agitated, confused or disoriented while in the hospital—even if it comes and goes, a common feature of hospital-induced delirium—alert the staff and ask specifically for a delirium evaluation from a mental health care provider. Basic treatment, including making sure the patient is well hydrated and nourished…stops taking dangerous medications if possible…gets daily exercise…is surrounded by familiar objects…and stays connected to family and friends, can often turn incipient delirium around before it gets too bad.

Did You Have a Heart Attack—And Not Know It?

Wilbert Aronow, MD, professor of medicine in the divisions of cardiology, geriatrics and pulmonary/critical medicine, and chief of the cardiology clinic at Westchester Medical Center/New York Medical College in Valhalla, New York.

When you have a heart attack, you know it because the main symptom—crushing chest pain—is overwhelmingly obvious. That's what most of us believe about heart attacks. But it's not always true.

What few people realize: Studies show that 20% to 60% of all heart attacks in people over age 45 are unrecognized or "silent." And the older you are, the more likely it is that you've already had a silent heart attack. In a study of 110 people with a mean age of 82, an astounding 68% had suffered a silent heart attack.

What happens during a silent heart attack? You may have no symptoms at all. Or you may have symptoms that are so mild—for example, a bout of breathlessness, digestive upset or neurological symptoms such as fainting—that neither you nor your doctor connects them with a heart attack.

Scientists don't know why some people have unrecognized heart attacks. But they do know that a silent heart attack is a real heart attack and can cause as much damage to heart muscle as a nonsilent heart attack. And just like a person with a known heart attack, anyone who has had a silent heart attack is at higher risk for another heart attack, heart failure, stroke...or sudden death from an irregular heartbeat.

Recent scientific evidence: In a six-year study by cardiologists from the University of California in San Diego and San Francisco—published in *Clinical Research in Cardiology*—people who were diagnosed with a silent heart attack at the beginning of the study were 80% more likely to have another "cardiovascular event," such as a heart attack or stroke, by the end of the study period.

In a five-year study by cardiologists at the Mayo Clinic, people with an unrecognized heart attack were seven times more likely to die of heart disease than people who didn't have an unrecognized heart attack.

If you have risk factors for heart disease, it is vitally important to your health that you find out if you have had a silent heart attack. *Here's how...*

THE KEY TO DETECTION

If you're at high risk for heart disease, your primary care physician should perform an electrocardiogram (EKG)—a test that checks for problems with the electrical activity of your heart—every year during your regular checkup. If the EKG reveals significant "Q-waves"—markers of damaged heart tissue—you have had a silent heart attack.

"High risk" means that you have two or more risk factors for heart disease. These risk factors include a family history of heart disease (in a first-degree relative such as a sibling or parent)...high blood pressure...smoking...inactivity...obesity...high LDL "bad" cholesterol...low HDL "good" cholesterol...high triglycerides...and type 2 diabetes.

The groups at highest risk for having an unrecognized heart attack are adults over age 65...women...and people of any age with type 2 diabetes.

THE TREATMENT YOU NEED

If your EKG reveals a previously unrecognized heart attack, it's wise to see a cardiologist and receive the exact same treatment that you would get if you had a recognized heart attack. *Elements of that treatment should include...*

•**Treadmill stress test.** The cardiologist will check for and interpret many variables, such as your symptoms (if any), the electrical patterns of your heart rhythms and your blood pressure while you are on a treadmill.

Important: Be sure to get your cardiologist's advice on special steps to take to ensure accurate results. For example, you should have no caffeine within 24 hours of the test.

If the results of the stress test indicate "severe myocardial ischemia"—poor blood flow to the heart muscle—it may be necessary to have a coronary angiogram (X-rays of the heart's arteries) to accurately diagnose the degree of blockage and decide whether you should pursue such options as angioplasty (in which a balloon is inserted into the coronary artery and inflated to restore normal blood flow) or coronary bypass surgery (in which a blood vessel is grafted from another part of the body to give blood a new pathway to the heart).

However, in most cases, heart disease that is associated with a silent heart attack can be managed with such as not smoking...losing weight if you're overweight...and getting regular exercise. *In addition, medications may include…*

- **Aspirin.** A daily dose of 81 mg of aspirin is the best choice for an antiplatelet drug to reduce the risk for blood clots.

Very important: A higher dose does not increase the cardiovascular benefit—but does increase the risk for gastrointestinal bleeding.

- **Beta-blocker.** This class of drugs slows the heart rate, relaxing the heart and helping to manage high blood pressure.

- **Angiotensin-converting enzyme (ACE) inhibitor.** These drugs expand blood vessels, improving blood flow and lowering blood pressure—thus allowing the heart to work less.

- **Statin.** If you have heart disease, this cholesterol-lowering medication reduces your risk for another heart attack or dying from heart disease—regardless of whether your levels of LDL "bad" cholesterol are high or low.

In addition, statin use should be accompanied by a diet that is low in cholesterol (less than 200 mg per day) and low in saturated fat (less than 7% of total calories).

Also important: It's crucial that people with diabetes maintain tight control of their HbA1C levels. This measure of long-term blood sugar control should be less than 7%.

However, HbA1C levels should not be aggressively lowered below 6.5% in diabetes patients with cardiovascular disease, according to the Action to Control Cardiovascular Risk in Diabetes study—that increases the risk for death because it would indicate that blood glucose is at times too low.

In general, the best way for people with diabetes to protect against heart attacks and strokes is to give up cigarettes if they smoke… lose weight if necessary…reduce blood pressure to 130–139/80–89 mmHg…and reduce LDL cholesterol to less than 70 mg/dL.

If these lifestyle measures do not also sufficiently lower the person's HbA1C level, standard antidiabetes medication can be used.

Medical Tests That Can Cause More Harm Than Good

Reid B. Blackwelder, MD, FAAFP, president of the American Academy of Family Physicians. He is also a practicing family physician in Johnson City, Tennessee, and professor of family medicine at Quillen College of Medicine at East Tennessee State University, also in Johnson City.

Are you getting cookie-cutter medical care? Too many people are—and one glaring example of this is the number of tests and procedures that are being prescribed regardless of the individual's specific health situation.

In fact, there's more and more evidence that many of the tests that are given so routinely are causing more harm than good.

Here are some popular tests that are often not necessary…*

CT SCANS FOR LOW-BACK PAIN

If your low back is giving you fits, your doctor may order an X-ray or even a more detailed test such as a CT scan to see what's going on.

Problem: Americans are receiving doses of radiation from X-rays and CT scans (not to mention spending enormous amounts of money) to diagnose a problem that will likely go away on its own in a few weeks. In some cases, an incidental finding that's not even related to the pain leads to unnecessary back surgery.

Unless you are experiencing worsening nerve damage (such as loss of bladder or bowel control or loss of sensation or muscle power in your legs) or have cancer (which could possibly spread to the back), you probably don't need an imaging test within the first six weeks of your back pain.

Also: There is no medical or legal reason to get X-rays as a "baseline" for work-related back injuries.

*The tests in this article are evaluated at *ChoosingWisely.org*, a website that advises patients and doctors on a wide range of tests and procedures. Developed by more than 50 medical specialty societies, such as the American Academy of Family Physicians and the American College of Surgeons, the information is based on the most current scientific evidence. Remember to check with your doctor for advice that's tailored to your specific needs.

BONE-DENSITY TESTS

For years, physicians have been routinely recommending bone-density tests using dual-energy X-ray absorptiometry (DXA). The test estimates the amount of bone in the hip and spine, which is a marker for osteoporosis. Until recently, women have often been advised to have a "baseline" DXA screening at menopause…then periodically after that.

Problem: Being labeled with "preosteoporosis" (commonly known as osteopenia) can start you on a medical journey of repeated DXA testing and use of medications that may be harmful. For example, osteoporosis drugs known as *bisphosphonates—risedronate* (Actonel), *ibandronate* (Boniva) and *alendronate* (Fosamax)—have been shown, in rare cases, to cause an unusual fracture of the thigh bone when one of these medications is taken for longer than five years.

And evidence shows that this test is not always a reliable predictor of fractures even in high-risk patients who are already receiving drug therapy for osteoporosis.

New thinking: Unless you are a woman age 65 or older or a man age 70 or older—or you have a special risk factor for osteoporosis, such as family history, smoking or alcohol abuse or use of corticosteroid drugs—you probably don't need DXA screening.

If your DXA test results show that you have normal bone mass, you don't need to be tested again for up to 10 years, provided you don't break a bone or show other signs of osteoporosis, such as losing more than an inch in height.

CAROTID ARTERY IMAGING

Your carotid arteries carry blood from your heart through the neck to your brain. If those arteries become narrowed from a buildup of plaque (a condition known as carotid artery stenosis, or CAS), your blood flow is slowed and your risk for stroke increases. Doctors can use ultrasound, magnetic resonance angiography (MRA) or computed tomography angiography (CTA) scans to check for plaque in these arteries.

Problem: If testing does show a blockage, you may be advised to take medication that won't necessarily improve your life expectancy. You may even be urged to undergo surgery (endarterectomy) to clear the artery. However, this is a difficult and complex operation that in rare cases leads to stroke, heart attack or even death.

New thinking: Unless you are experiencing symptoms, such as stroke, transient ischemic attack (a so-called "mini-stroke") or unexplained dizziness, you probably do not need to be screened for CAS. Evidence shows that the harms of screening (and subsequent treatment) in people without symptoms usually outweigh the benefits.

If you do undergo screening for CAS, surgery is generally not recommended unless you have more than 70% blockage in one or both of your carotid arteries and you have had a stroke or ministroke in the previous six months.

EKG AND STRESS TEST

During your routine physical, your doctor may have ordered an electrocardiogram (EKG or ECG) to measure your heart's electrical activity and/or a cardiac stress test to check the same functions but under conditions where you are "stressed" via exercise or medication.

Problem: Unnecessary stress testing can lead to false-positive tests—indicating that something is wrong when you are actually healthy. This can mean more follow-up tests, including CT scans or coronary angiography, both of which expose you to radiation. And in rare cases, an angiography actually leads to a heart attack in people who have the test. Sometimes, after a "bad" EKG or stress test, a doctor may also prescribe unnecessary heart medication.

New thinking: If you don't have any heart-related symptoms (such as chest pain or shortness of breath), the evidence shows that an annual EKG or other cardiac screening is unlikely to prevent a heart attack, catch a hidden heart problem or otherwise make you any healthier than you already are.

If you are getting noncardiac thoracic surgery (for example, on the lungs, esophagus or other organs in the chest), you do not need to have stress testing before the operation unless you have a history of heart problems. In healthy patients, testing rarely changes how they are treated, so it's generally not necessary.

The Generic-Drug Rip-Off

David Belk, MD, a physician based in Alameda, California, specializing in internal medicine. He is founder of the True Cost of Healthcare blog, which provides information about health-care cost and billing issues. TrueCostOfHealthCare.net

Using health insurance to fill a prescription for a generic drug could dramatically increase your out-of-pocket costs, particularly if you have not yet reached your policy's annual deductible. That's because people who use health insurance have to pay the price that the insurance company has set for the drug, and with generic drugs, these prices often are much higher than the prices you might pay when no insurance is used—sometimes hundreds of dollars higher for a 90-day supply.

Here's what happens behind the scenes: Many generic drugs cost pharmacies 10 cents a pill or less. A value-oriented pharmacy, such as those at Costco, Walmart and Kroger, or a reputable online pharmacy, such as Health-Warehouse.com, might charge as little as $4 for a 30-day supply or $10 for a 90-day supply—if you don't use insurance. What's more, even after you reach your deductible, many insurance policies require a co-pay that is higher than what these types of pharmacies charge for generic drugs.

Among the many widely used drugs that can be purchased without insurance as generics for as little as $10 for a 90-day supply are the blood pressure medications *atenolol, carvedilol, clonidine* and *furosemide*…blood-clot-prevention drug *warfarin*…diabetes drugs *glimepiride, glipizide, glyburide* and *metformin*…cholesterol medication *lovastatin*…antibiotic *amoxicillin*…and pain medication *naproxen*.

What to do: When filling a prescription for a generic drug, check whether it's cheaper to fill the prescription without using your coverage. Also, ask pharmacies whether they have a membership or rewards program that can further reduce the cost. Use GoodRx.com to comparative shop local prescription prices.

On the other hand, if you expect to spend a lot more than your deductible for medical costs in a given year, it might make sense to pay the higher prices so that you get past the deductible period more quickly. In some cases, depending on the specifics of your coverage, that might result in greater overall savings.

3

Doctor-Tested Home Remedies for Everything from Hiccups to Hemorrhoids

Pinch Here...Poke There...17 Natural Remedies You Always Have with You

Here are 17 remedies for common health problems that all have one thing in common— you always have these simple remedies with you!

•**Dry mouth.** When it's important for you to seem calm and sound confident, don't let your dry mouth get in the way. Gently chew on your tongue. Within about 30 seconds, you will manufacture all the saliva you need to end this uncomfortable condition. If people notice, they will just think that you're chewing gum or sucking a candy.

•**Burned fingertips.** If you get a minor burn on your fingertips, simply hold your earlobe—it's an acupressure point. Place your thumb on the back of the lobe and the burned fingertips on the front of the lobe. Stay that way for one minute. It works like magic to relieve the pain.

•**Hiccups.** *Here are two remedies...*

•Pretend that your finger is a mustache. Place it under your nose, and press in hard for 30 seconds. That should do it, but if not...

•Take a deep breath. Without letting any air out, swallow. Breathe in a little bit more, then swallow. Keep inhaling and swallowing until you absolutely can't inhale or swallow anymore. Then, in a controlled way, slowly exhale.

•Motion sickness. Pull out and pinch the skin in the middle of your inner wrist, about one inch from your palm. Keep pulling and pinching, alternating wrists, until you feel better. It shouldn't take too long.

•**Leg cramps.** The second you get a cramp in your leg, "acupinch" it away. Use your thumb and your index finger to pinch your philtrum—the skin between your nose and

Lydia Wilen and Joan Wilen are folk-remedy experts based in New York City. They are coauthors of many books, including *Bottom Line's Household Magic* and *Secret Food Cures.*

upper lip. Pinch it for about 20 seconds until the pain and the cramp disappear.

• **Stomachache.** This remedy came to us from an Asian massage therapist. If you are having stomach discomfort, massage the acupressure points at the sides of your knees, just below the kneecaps. This will relieve your stomachache.

• **Warts.** First thing each morning, dab some of your own spittle on the wart (but do not lick the wart). "First thing" means before you brush your teeth. We don't know why it works—it just does.

• **Hemorrhoids.** Edgar Cayce, who is often called the father of holistic medicine, recommended this exercise for the treatment of hemorrhoids…

• Stand with your feet about six inches apart, hands at sides.

• Then raise your hands up to the ceiling, and if balance isn't a problem for you, gradually rise up on your toes at the same time.

• Bend forward, and bring your hands as close to the floor as you can get them.

• Go back to the first position, and do it again.

Perform this exercise for two or three minutes twice every day, one hour after breakfast and one hour after dinner, until your hemorrhoids are relieved.

• **Choking cough.** When you're not actually choking on something but you just are coughing as though you are, raise your hands as high as you can and the choking cough will stop.

• **Tension headache.** Tense all the muscles in your face, neck, jaw, scalp and shoulders. Hold that tension for at least 30 seconds. Then, suddenly, relax completely, letting go of all the tension, and your headache along with it.

• **Gas.** Try this yoga pose called the wind-relieving pose. Lie on your back with your legs and arms extended. As you exhale, draw both knees to your chest. Clasp your hands around them. While holding only your right knee with both hands, release your left leg and extend it along the floor. Hold this pose for one minute. Draw your left knee back in toward your chest, and clasp your hands around both knees

again. Then while holding only your left knee, release your right leg and extend it along the floor. Hold this pose for up to a minute. Finally, draw both knees to your chest. Then with an exhalation, release and extend both legs.

• **Fatigue.** If you are having a hard time staying awake or paying attention, here are five energizing strategies. *Try the one that is doable in your situation…*

• Chinese theory is that "tiredness" collects on the insides of your elbows and the backs of your knees. Wake up your body by slap-slap-slapping those areas.

• Run in place for about two minutes.

• Energy lines directly connected to internal organs and body functions run through your earlobes. Use your thumbs and index fingers to rub your earlobes for about 15 seconds. This should wake up your entire nervous system.

• This visualization exercise will help you overcome drowsiness. Sit back, close your eyes, and let all the air out of your lungs. Imagine a bright blue-white energizing light entering and filling your entire body as you inhale slowly through your nostrils. Then open your eyes. You will feel refreshed.

• Boost your energy by belting out a few bars of a favorite cheerful song. Inhale deeply as you sing to bring more energizing oxygen into your lungs and increase circulation in your body.

Don't Let Your Bladder Run Your Life!

Holly Lucille, ND, RN, naturopathic doctor based in West Hollywood, California. She is the author of *Creating and Maintaining Balance: A Woman's Guide to Safe, Natural Hormone Health* and serves on the Institute for Natural Medicine Board of Directors. DrHollyLucille. com

---

Men and women who scout out restrooms wherever they are may think that others don't have to worry so much about their bladders. But that's not true.

Eye-opening statistic: One in every five adults over age 40 has overactive bladder…and after the age of 65, a whopping one in every three adults is affected. If you regularly have a strong and sudden urge to urinate and/or need to hit the john eight or more times a day (or more than once at night), chances are you have the condition, too.

Postmenopausal women (due to their low estrogen levels) and men with enlarged prostate issues are at increased risk of having overactive bladder. Urinary tract infections, use of certain medications (such as antidepressants and drugs to treat high blood pressure and insomnia) and even constipation also can cause or worsen the condition.

But there is a bright side. Research is now uncovering several surprisingly simple natural approaches that are highly effective for many people with overactive bladder. *Among the best...*

START WITH YOUR DIET

Most people don't connect a bladder problem to their diets. But there is a strong link. *My advice...*

• **Take a hard line with irritants.** Alcohol, caffeine and artificial sweeteners can exacerbate the feeling of urgency caused by overactive bladder. Cutting back on these items is a good first step, but they often creep back into one's diet over time.

What helps: Keep it simple—completely avoid alcohol, caffeine (all forms, including coffee, tea and caffeine-containing foods such as chocolate) and artificial sweeteners. Stick to decaffeinated coffee and herbal teas, and use agave and stevia as sweeteners.

Many individuals also are sensitive to certain foods, such as corn, wheat, dairy, eggs and peanuts. They often trigger an immune reaction that contributes to overall inflammation in the body, including in the bladder. If your symptoms of urinary urgency and/or frequency increase after eating one of these (or any other) foods, your body may be having an inflammatory response that is also affecting your bladder. Eliminate these foods from your diet.

• **Keep your gut healthy.** The scientific evidence is still in the early stages, but research now suggests that leaky gut syndrome, in which excess bacterial or fungal growth harms the mucosal membrane in the intestines, is at the root of several health problems, including overactive bladder.

The theory is that an imbalance of microbes, a condition known as *dysbiosis*, can irritate the walls of the bladder just as it does in the gut.

What helps: Probiotics and oregano oil* capsules. Probiotics replenish "good" bacteria, and oregano oil has antibacterial properties that help cleanse "bad" bacteria and fungi from the gut.

• **Drink up!** People with overactive bladder often cut way back on their fluid intake because they already make so many trips to the bathroom. But when you don't drink enough fluids, urine tends to have an irritating effect because it becomes more concentrated. This increases urgency.

What helps: Drink half your body weight in ounces of water or herbal tea daily. Do not drink any fluids after 5 p.m. to help prevent bathroom runs during the night.

THE RIGHT SUPPLEMENTS

Cranberry supplements (or unsweetened cranberry juice) can be helpful for bladder infections, but they're usually not the best choice for overactive bladder. *My advice...*

• **Try pumpkin seed extract.** These capsules help tone and strengthen the tissue of your pelvic-floor muscles, which gives you better bladder control.

Typical dosage: 500 mg daily.

• **Consider *Angelica archangelica* extract.** This herb has gotten positive reviews from researchers who have investigated it as a therapy for overactive bladder.

Recent finding: When 43 men with overactive bladder took 300 mg of the herb daily, they made fewer trips to the bathroom. This study was about bladder capacity, not the prostate, so women can benefit, too.

Typical dosage: 100 mg daily.

*Talk to your doctor before trying any of these herbal remedies, especially if you take medication or have a chronic health condition. You may want to consult a naturopathic doctor. To find one near you, check *www. naturopathic.org.*

Easy Earache Remedy

Lydia Wilen and Joan Wilen are folk-remedy experts based in New York City. They are coauthors of many books, including *Bottom Line's Household Magic* and *Secret Food Cures*.

Is there a constant rumble of a leftover cold or flu in your ear? Earaches can be a sign of something serious, so don't turn a deaf ear if you have persistent, severe pain—see a doctor as soon as possible. But if you have a minor waterlogged feeling in your ear (and you recently had a cold or a bout of allergy symptoms), here's an easy, soothing home remedy to make this annoying condition disappear…

You'll need ginger and sesame oil (toasted or regular is fine…just make sure it's pure and not mixed with any other oil). Peel and slice a three-inch piece of ginger. Add to a small saucepan with one-half cup of water and bring to a boil, then simmer for 20 minutes (the water will reduce to about one-quarter cup). Let the ginger sit and steep and cool (a half hour or so should be enough). Add two teaspoons of the ginger water to two teaspoons of sesame oil, and stir well. With a clean eyedropper, drop two to three drops of this mixture into your ear and loosely plug with a cotton ball. (If some liquid leaks out, drop in a little more.) Relax with the cotton ball in your ear for at least an hour. Your ear should feel better soon after that.

Helpful hint: Since sesame oil can go rancid, be sure to store it in the refrigerator after opening. Just before using, let the refrigerated bottle sit on a warm stove top for a few minutes to thin the oil out a bit.

No More Neck Pain!

Robert Turner, PT, OCS, a board-certified orthopedic clinical specialist and clinical supervisor at the Hospital for Special Surgery's Spine Therapy Center in New York City. Turner is also a licensed acupuncturist and certified Pilates instructor.

Neck pain can be agonizing. But there's more at stake than the discomfort itself. This common complaint also can lead to collateral damage that you'd never expect—by contributing to anxiety or depression.

Problem: Far too many people live with this painful condition for years because they don't really get to the root of the problem.

What's the cause of all this pain? Much of it boils down to poor posture—we sit at computers or in cars for hours at a time…our heads leaning forward to help us see the screen or the road. With our arms extended in front of us, we naturally round forward and our chests tighten, weakening the back muscles—a significant but under-appreciated cause of neck pain.

If you hold a phone between your ear and shoulder or carry a heavy bag over one shoulder, you're only making matters worse. Or you may awaken with a "crick" in your neck from sleeping in an awkward position. And if you lie on the couch for hours at a time, you're speeding the muscle atrophy and inflexibility that will keep you in misery.

But there is hope! Doing the right type of stretching is incredibly effective at relieving neck pain.

What gets overlooked: While you might be tempted to target only the neck itself in these stretches, it's crucial to also do chest and back stretches to help correct musculoskeletal system imbalances and restore flexibility.

Here are four great stretches for neck pain—the entire routine can be performed in about 10 minutes.* (If you're short on time, just do the first two stretches when you start to feel neck discomfort or after you've been sitting for 90 minutes.)

• **Chicken wings.** This move opens the chest and strengthens the shoulder blades, which helps relieve pressure on the neck.

What to do: While sitting up straight on a chair, extend your arms out to the sides and touch your fingertips to your shoulders. Roll both shoulders back and down. You should feel the muscles between your blades contract. The key is not working too

*These exercises are safe for most people. If you experience pain, numbness or tingling in the hand or arm that does not go away after exercise or becomes worse, don't do the exercise again and tell your doctor.

hard—give it 50% of your effort, not 100%—or you'll end up straining your neck. Hold for one breath in and one breath out, then relax. Repeat 10 times. Perform this series twice a day.

•**Triple neck stretch.** These exercises stretch the larger muscles that attach the head and neck to the shoulders.

What to do: While sitting on the edge of a chair, lightly press the back of your right hand against the middle of your lower back, with your right elbow pointing directly out to the side. While look-

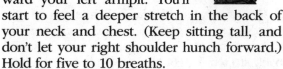

ing straight ahead, tilt your head to the left, being careful not to rotate your neck. (You can use your left hand to gently pull your head down, intensifying the stretch.) Hold for five to 10 breaths.

For the second step, with your right hand still on your back and your head still tilted to the left, rotate your chin down so that your nose is pointing toward your left armpit. You'll start to feel a deeper stretch in the back of your neck and chest. (Keep sitting tall, and don't let your right shoulder hunch forward.) Hold for five to 10 breaths.

Lastly, with your nose still pointing toward your armpit, place the palm of your right hand behind your neck, keeping your shoulder blades down, and hold for five to 10 breaths. Repeat the three-step series on the other side of your body, and you have just completed one round. Try to do one or two more rounds throughout the day...or whenever pain crops up.

•**Prone extension.** This move strengthens your back muscles so that your neck does not have to work so hard to maintain proper posture.

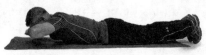

Note: If you have low-back pain, put a pillow under your hips when doing this stretch and the next one to avoid straining this part of your back.

What to do: Lie on your stomach on a padded mat or carpet with your hands stacked beneath your forehead, legs straight and your knees and ankles together.

Pull your navel in toward your spine to help support your lower back, and push both shoulder blades down toward your feet as you inhale and arch your upper back at least two to three inches off the floor (your hands and arms should rise with your upper body). Exhale on the way back down. Repeat for a total of 10 lifts. Take a brief break, then repeat two more sets, eventually progressing to three sets of 15.

•**Shoulder blade lift.** This stretch will strengthen the back and shoulder muscles that help maintain correct head and neck alignment.

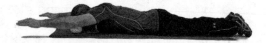

What to do: Lie on your stomach on a padded mat or carpet with a rolled-up towel placed beneath your forehead, nose pointing toward the floor to keep your neck in a straight line and your arms pointed forward in a Y formation.

While keeping your head down and neck relaxed, inhale as you lift your arms, hands and upper chest a few inches off the floor... hold for a beat, and exhale as your arms lower back down. Repeat 10 times. You will feel the muscles around the shoulder blades and middle back engage to lift the arms.

Caution: If you experience shoulder pain, modify the stretch by bending your elbows into a wide goalpost position. People who have had rotator cuff surgery or a shoulder injury can try this move while lying facedown on a bed, raising the arms off the edge of the bed toward the ceiling.

Easy Home Remedy to Stop a Cold Sore

About 85% of all Americans are prone to cold sores. These unsightly blemishes are caused by the herpes simplex virus. They often burst into view when you least want them—usually when your resistance is low because of a cold, the flu, pregnancy, sunburn, or before a job interview, your wedding day or some other stressful event. Cold sores generally take about two weeks to clear up. *Here's an easy home remedy to speed up the healing process…*

Combine one teaspoon of apple cider vinegar with one tablespoon of honey (preferably raw honey), and dab the cold sore with a cotton swab dipped in this mixture. Do this three times a day (once in the morning, afternoon and evening). The sore should be gone in less than a week.

Lydia Wilen and Joan Wilen are are folk-remedy experts based in New York City. They are coauthors of many books, including *Bottom Line's Household Magic* and *Secret Food Cures.*

Tart Cherries Before Your Trip

Natural jet-lag remedy: Tart cherries. They have high levels of melatonin, which helps regulate your circadian rhythm and induce sleepiness.

Best: Have one-half cup of dried tart cherries (such as Montmorency) or two tablespoons of any cherry juice concentrate one hour before you wish to sleep on the plane and an hour before bedtime for the three days after you land.

Russel Reiter, PhD, professor of neuroendocrinology, University of Texas Health Science Center, San Antonio.

Natural Remedy for Irritable Bowel Syndrome (IBS)

Peppermint oil can alleviate the gastrointestinal symptoms associated with IBS, including flatulence and abdominal pain and distension, by blocking the flow of calcium into muscle cells in the intestines, which in turn reduces muscle contractions.

Best: When symptoms are present, take two coated capsules of peppermint oil three times daily.

Alexander Ford, MD, senior lecturer, section of molecular gastroenterology, Leeds Institute of Molecular Medicine, Leeds University, UK.

Natural Remedy for Anxiety

The light, soothing fragrance of lavender oil has long been used in aromatherapy to ease anxiety and insomnia. Lavender oil supplements are also available for anxiety. For example, Calm Aid by Nature's Way contains Silexan, a type of lavender oil shown in clinical studies to ease anxiety as effectively as the benzodiazepine drug *lorazepam* (Ativan). Those who took the supplement also reported better sleep quality. I recommend taking one 80-mg softgel in the morning with a glass of water. Side effects are rare but can include nausea, constipation and headache. Check with your doctor before trying.

Holly Lucille, ND, RN, naturopathic doctor based in West Hollywood, California. DrHollyLucille.com

Natural Remedies for Four Very Common Health Problems

Laurie Steelsmith, ND, a naturopathic doctor and acupuncturist in private practice in Honolulu. She is the author of *Natural Choices for Women's Health.* NaturalChoicesforWomen.com

Chances are you have at least one health problem that you experience regularly—perhaps insomnia, constipation, urinary tract infections or another ailment. While it is tempting to pop a pill and hope that whatever it is will go away, that recurring problem is your body's way of telling you that something is out of balance.

Here are five common complaints and how you can treat the underlying causes using natural, common-sense remedies. All of the supplements mentioned here are sold in health-food stores and are safe for most women—but check with your doctor before taking any new supplements.

ENERGY SWINGS

What it could mean: Too many ups and downs in energy generally point to a diet that is too high in simple carbohydrates—such as white potatoes, white rice, white flour and refined sugar—and too low in fiber and lean protein. With little to slow digestion, your body rapidly processes a meal or snack of simple carbohydrates (such as pancakes and hash browns), causing your blood sugar levels to spike and then quickly crash. *Self-defense...*

• **Eat whole grains instead of simple carbohydrates**—brown rice instead of white rice... oatmeal with fresh fruit instead of a sugary breakfast cereal...popcorn instead of potato chips. The additional fiber prolongs digestion and makes your blood sugar levels less prone to fast-paced highs and lows.

• **Eat more lean protein**—from skinless chicken, lean beef and cold-water fish (such as salmon and mackerel), tofu and beans—which helps to stabilize blood sugar levels.

Helpful: Choose organic poultry, meat and wild fish rather than most farm-raised fish to minimize exposure to environmental toxins, such as pesticides and herbicides.

INSOMNIA

What it could mean: Low levels of progesterone, a hormone that has a calming effect. High anxiety levels also may contribute to your sleeplessness.

Self-defense: Try one or more of the following sleep inducers...

• **Help your body to produce more serotonin, a brain chemical that affects mood.** Supplement with 5-HTP, a derivative of the amino acid tryptophan, which the body uses to manufacture serotonin. Start at 100 milli-

grams (mg), taken once daily before bed, and work up to 500 mg over two weeks.

Caution: Don't use 5-HTP if you're taking a selective serotonin reuptake inhibitor (SSRI) antidepressant, such as *Prozac, Zoloft* or *Paxil.*

• **Reduce anxiety.** Supplement with L-theanine, an amino acid derived from green tea that can produce a noticeable calming effect within 30 minutes of ingestion. Take 200 mg every night at bedtime...and again if you wake up in the middle of the night.

• **Increase your progesterone.** If you're still menstruating each month, you also can talk to your doctor about applying natural progesterone cream—enough to provide approximately 25 mg of progesterone (about one-quarter teaspoon)—each night for 14 nights from mid-cycle until your period starts. If you are postmenopausal, you can apply the progesterone cream for 21 days of the month, then take seven days off.

Note: Possible side effects include nausea, headaches and diarrhea.

DIARRHEA OR CONSTIPATION

What it could mean: A diet high in simple carbohydrates may lead to the overgrowth of "unfriendly" bacteria in the digestive tract... and the imbalance can progress into irritable bowel syndrome, a common condition characterized by diarrhea, constipation or both. *Self-defense...*

• **Eliminate simple carbohydrates from your diet**—such as refined sugar, beer, white flour and white potatoes—and eat more vegetables, lean organic protein and fiber-rich beans, brown rice and whole-wheat bread.

• **Eradicate unfriendly bacteria. If your symptoms are mild, take garlic**—the herb's natural antifungal and antibacterial properties target unwelcome residents of your digestive tract. The first week, eat one clove of raw garlic once a day, or take one 900-mg garlic tablet twice a day. Starting the second week, eat two cloves of raw garlic a day, or take one 900-mg garlic tablet two or three times a day. Continue this regimen until symptoms subside.

Note: Take garlic with meals to avoid stomach upset. To prevent bad breath, use garlic tablets labeled "odorless" or "sociable" and/or eat fresh parsley after taking the garlic.

• **Supplement with probiotics.** Two weeks after the garlic treatment is finished, restore balance to your digestive tract by adding "friendly" bacteria. Take a probiotic supplement that provides a total of one billion live organisms per day for at least one month.

Recommended probiotic brands: Natren and Theralac.

CHRONIC YEAST INFECTIONS

What it could mean: Overgrowth of yeast in your digestive tract may cause an overgrowth of yeast in your vagina. Often this is triggered by eating too much sugar—yeast's favorite meal. *Self-defense…*

• **Cut off yeast's food supply.** Follow the previous diet recommendations given for diarrhea or constipation.

• **Use a tea tree oil–based douche to target vaginal yeast.**

Note: Do this only if you know you have a yeast infection. Make your own douche by adding 10 drops of tea tree oil to one pint of water. Using a douche bag (sold at drugstores), douche while sitting on the toilet or standing in the shower twice a day for one week.

• **Reduce unfriendly bacteria and yeast throughout your body.** Take a probiotic supplement that provides one billion live organisms daily for at least one month.

URINARY TRACT INFECTIONS

What it could mean: Dehydration, excessive stress or a low estrogen level due to menopause can allow bacteria to take up residence in the urinary tract. *Self-defense…*

• **Drink water.** Aim for at least 48 ounces of filtered water daily to encourage the elimination of bacteria from the urinary tract.

• **Empty your bladder as soon as you feel the urge** and as completely as possible to evacuate bacteria before they can thrive.

• **Drink 10 ounces of unsweetened cranberry juice daily** to prevent bacteria from at-taching to the lining of the urethra (the tube that empties urine from the bladder).

Also: You can take six cranberry capsules daily instead of juice, or follow the label for cranberry extract.

• **Boost your estrogen levels.** If the problem persists, speak to your doctor about using a low-dose prescription vaginal estrogen cream, which strengthens the tissue of the vulva and urethra, making you more resistant to infection.

A Drug-Free Solution to a Lingering Cough

Study titled "Honey plus coffee versus systemic steroid in the treatment of persistent post-infectious cough: a randomized controlled trial," published in *Primary Care Respiratory Journal.*

A very common cause of a lingering cough is an upper respiratory infection that has come and gone. You and your doctor may run a gamut—and run up a huge medical bill—in search of an exotic, life-threatening cause of a die-hard cough that's really happening because cough-triggering nerves have become overly irritated and hypersensitive from that cold you had.

Nature's cure for an aggravating cough is honey, of course, but it still might not be a match for a cough that has lingered for weeks. Well, adding just a little bit of a certain beloved beverage to a spoonful of honey could kick honey's cough-soothing properties up a notch. In fact, the combination may be so potent that it not only knocks out a persistent cough, it prevents a horrid mouth and throat condition common to people receiving chemotherapy.

It turns out that having some coffee with your honey (instead of the other way around) does the trick.

HOMEMADE COUGH RELIEF

A team of Iranian researchers ran across this seeming marvel when they compared a honey-coffee remedy with a steroid solution and an expectorant cough suppressant. They performed the comparison in 97 adults whose cough had lingered for more than three weeks after a respiratory infection came and went. Smokers and any other potential study participants whose coughs could be diagnosed as something other than a "persistent post-infectious cough" were not allowed to participate in the study.

Participants were divided into three groups. One group received a "jam" made of honey and coffee (the honey-to-coffee ratio was about five parts honey to one part instant coffee). Another group received a jam containing the steroid prednisolone, which is sometimes prescribed to people with persistent cough... and the third group received a jam containing guaifenesin—the active ingredient in expectorants such as Mucinex and Robitussin. All three remedies were made by a pharmacist to look and taste the same by adding food coloring, coffee essence, artificial honey flavor and liquid glucose to the products containing the steroid and expectorant.

The participants drank one tablespoon of their jam dissolved in about seven ounces of warm water three times per day (every eight hours) for a week. All of the participants knew what remedies were being compared, but none knew which one he or she was taking. And they all agreed not to use any other anti-inflammatory drugs or cough suppressants or otherwise consume any honey or coffee during the study.

Results: The honey and coffee combo strongly beat out the steroid, with the combo reducing cough frequency by 93% compared with 20% for the steroid. And it obliterated the expectorant cough suppressant, which had virtually no effect on the frequency of persistent cough.

STUMBLING ON ANOTHER REMEDY

When the researchers noticed that the honey-coffee remedy healed the irritated throats of their study participants very quickly, a bright idea occurred to them. They turned their sights to studying the combo in people with mucositis, a condition affecting 40% of people receiving chemotherapy, 80% receiving radiotherapy of the head and neck and all patients who undergo bone marrow transplantation.

In mucositis, raw, ulcerous, burning sores develop in the mouth, throat and sometimes other parts of the digestive tract. This happens because cancer therapies target all fast-growing cells whether they are healthy or not. These include cells lining the mouth, throat, stomach and intestines.

The research team designed a study similar to the cough study, but in this case pitted a honey/instant coffee syrup against a steroid syrup and a plain honey syrup (all flavored to taste the same).

Results were equally remarkable—symptoms improved by 86% in the coffee/honey group...by 64% in the honey-only group...and by only 43% in the steroid group.

Coffee and honey—who would've thought?!

The researchers theorized that the antioxidant, anti-inflammatory and salivary-gland-stimulating effects of honey and the antioxidant effects of coffee had a synergistically protective effect on mucous membranes of the mouth and throat.

This study (like the one on lingering cough) did not comment on safety or side effects. Patients in the mucositis study were instructed to sip three teaspoons of syrup every three hours—that's about nine tablespoons of diluted honey and coffee per day—that doesn't sound too good for blood sugar levels or the waistline. Still, it might be a lesser evil compared with mucositis and its complications, which include infection of mouth and throat sores that can lead to life-threatening sepsis.

Also, although steroids are sometimes used in other parts of the world to treat mucositis, they're not used for this in the United States. Here, treatment of severe mucositis involves drugs that aid cell growth or else cryotherapy, which freezes away damaged sore-causing cells. Patients are also instructed to frequently brush their teeth to thwart bacterial growth and gargle with salty water and/or baking soda three to four times per day to keep mucous membranes moist and clean. They may also be told to use mouth- and throat-coating products that reduce pain (oral products that contain lidocaine, for example) and soothe the affected area (products such as Kaopectate).

That said, steroids are sometimes used here in America to treat serious cases of canker sores or other types of mouth ulcers and inflammation, such as those caused by allergic reactions.

The Iranian researchers' use of a steroid in their study of mucositis may not have been in line with American standards, but that doesn't seem to take away from the fact that their honey and coffee concoction had an impressive effect on symptoms of mucositis and mouth sores—as it did on relieving a persistent cough.

WORTH A TRY?

If a lingering cough that set in after a cold is driving you crazy (or if you are predisposed to mouth and throat irritation or are receiving chemotherapy or radiotherapy), this coffee-honey concoction might be worth a try. If your doctor gives you the green light (as in, a frequent daily dosage of caffeine/honey is OK for your blood sugar levels), then try this at home: Mix one-half teaspoon of instant coffee granules with two-and-a-half teaspoons of honey. Stir into seven ounces of warm water. Drink three servings a day.

The Simple 25¢ Remedy —A Quick Fix for Pain

Burton S. Schuler, DPM, podiatrist and director of the Ambulatory Foot Clinic at the Podiatric Pain Management Center in Panama City, Florida. He is author of *Why You Really Hurt*. FootCare4u.com

Millions of Americans live with chronic pain in their backs, hips, legs and feet. Many self-medicate with ibuprofen or other analgesics…or they undergo batteries of expensive tests to identify the underlying problem.

Do this first: Take off your socks and look at your toes. If the second toe is even slightly longer than the big toe, you might have Morton's toe, a condition that disrupts normal alignment and can cause pain throughout the body, particularly in the back, legs and feet.

The condition is named after Dudley J. Morton, MD, of Yale Medical School, who first wrote about it causing foot problems. Janet Travell, MD—White House physician to former presidents Kennedy and Johnson—took the concept further by explaining that Morton's toe could cause pain all over the body.

It's estimated that up to 15% of Americans have Morton's toe. Among those with chronic musculoskeletal pain, the prevalence might be as high as 80%. People are born with Morton's toe, but it usually takes decades of accumulated stress and the age-related loss of tissue elasticity to start producing symptoms that can develop into chronic pain.

WHY IT HURTS

When we walk and our feet push off from the ground, the big toe typically touches before the other toes. For a fraction of a second, it absorbs virtually all of the body's weight. Then as the foot rolls forward, some of the pressure is shifted to the adjoining, weaker toes.

In patients with Morton's toe, the first metatarsal bone (in the big toe) is abnormally short and the longer second metatarsal bone typically touches the ground first and absorbs most of the body's weight. The second metatarsal bone isn't strong enough for this much pressure. To compensate, the foot overpronates—it rolls in the direction of the big toe to support the excess weight.

Overpronation makes the foot unstable. It also prevents the big toe from pushing your weight upward. This means that other muscles and joints have to compensate.

The result: Decades of abnormal stress that can disrupt your posture and potentially damage joints throughout the body, causing pain.

THE 25¢ FIX

The simple, inexpensive remedy for Morton's toe is a toe pad. It will act like a shim under the first metatarsal bone and cause the big toe to meet the ground a fraction of a second sooner. This will prevent overpronation and help keep the foot stable. It often relieves symptoms within a few weeks—and sometimes right away.

Exception: Because a toe pad changes the body's alignment, some people experience a temporary increase in pain. This usually diminishes within a few days.

Once the pain goes away, you still will need to wear a toe pad every day, just as someone with sight problems needs to wear glasses or contact lenses every day. *To make a toe pad...*

•**Buy a package of inexpensive foam shoe inserts.** I have found that Dr. Scholl's Molefoam is a good product for making a toe pad (one pack provides six to eight toe pads). Just about any product will work—even no-name brands available at most pharmacies and discount stores, usually for less than $2.

Cut out a rectangle about one-inch wide and two-and-a-half inches long. That's about the size of a stick of chewing gum or a Band-Aid. Put it over the first metatarsal head, the bulge on the bottom of the foot that is below the point where the big toe joins the foot. Position the pad so that the longer dimension runs lengthwise with the foot. If the insole doesn't have an adhesive backing, tape it to the foot with duct tape, electrical tape or even Scotch tape. It does not have to look pretty.

You can take the toe pad off at night and put it back on the foot in the morning. One toe pad usually lasts two to four days.

Helpful: If you don't have a foam insert, a quarter can work. Anything that adds thickness to the first metatarsal head will help restore proper alignment.

APPLY HEAT

If a toe pad doesn't eliminate the pain right away, you might want to apply heat. Rest your feet on a heating pad or soak them in warm water for about 15 minutes, once or twice a day.

If after two to three weeks you still have pain, see your physician.

Pick Up a Broom to Stay Healthy!

A clean house and well-maintained property were key indicators of well-being, according to an analysis of more than 300 adults over age 65 with at least one chronic illness. In fact, they were more important than other factors, such as education, income and neighborhood.

Possible explanation: Living in an orderly environment requires a certain amount of physical exercise as well as cognitive skills.

Kathy D. Wright, PhD, RN, researcher, Case Western Reserve University, Cleveland.

4

Keep Your Mind Razor-Sharp for Life!

Dr. Kosik's Alzheimer's Prevention Plan

If someone told you that there was a pill with no side effects and strong evidence showing that it helps prevent Alzheimer's disease, would you take it? Of course, you would!

The truth is, there's no such "magic bullet," but most adults do have the ability to dramatically decrease their risk for this dreaded disease.

A window of opportunity: According to the latest scientific evidence, slowing or blocking Alzheimer's plaques (buildups of dangerous protein fragments), which are now known to develop years before memory loss and other symptoms are noticeable, could be the key to stopping this disease.

Dr. Kenneth S. Kosik, a renowned neuroscientist who has researched Alzheimer's for 25 years, *shared with us the habits that he incorporates into his daily routine to help prevent Alzheimer's...*

STEP 1: **Make exercise exciting.** You may know that frequent exercise—particularly aerobic exercise, which promotes blood flow to the brain—is the most effective Alzheimer's prevention strategy. Unfortunately, many people become bored and stop exercising.

Scientific evidence: Because exercise raises levels of brain-derived neurotrophic factor, it promotes the growth of new brain cells and may help prevent shrinkage of the hippocampus (a part of the brain involved in memory).

What I do: Most days, I spend 35 minutes on an elliptical trainer, followed by some weight training (increasing muscle mass helps prevent diabetes—an Alzheimer's risk factor). To break up the monotony, I go mountain biking on sunny days. I advise patients who have trouble sticking to an exercise regimen to try

Kenneth S. Kosik, MD, the Harriman Professor of Neuroscience Research and codirector of the Neuroscience Research Institute at the University of California, Santa Barbara, where he specializes in the causes and treatments of neurodegeneration, particularly Alzheimer's disease. Dr. Kosik is coauthor of *Outsmarting Alzheimer's.* KennethSKosikMD.com out the new virtual-reality equipment available in many gyms. While riding a stationary bike, for example, you can watch a monitor that puts you in the Tour de France!

Also helpful: To keep your exercise regimen exciting, go dancing. A recent 20-year study found that dancing reduced dementia risk more than any other type of exercise—perhaps because many types of dancing (such as tango, salsa and Zumba) involve learning new steps and aerobic activity. Do the type of dancing that appeals to you most.

STEP 2: Keep your eating plan simple. A nutritious diet is important for Alzheimer's prevention, but many people assume that they'll have to make massive changes, so they get overwhelmed and don't even try. To avoid this trap, keep it simple—all healthful diets have a few common elements, including an emphasis on antioxidant-rich foods (such as fruit and vegetables)…not too much red meat…and a limited amount of processed foods that are high in sugar, fat or additives.

Scientific evidence: Research has shown that people who consume more than four daily servings of vegetables have a 40% lower rate of cognitive decline than those who get less than one daily serving.

What I do: I try to eat more vegetables, particularly broccoli, cauliflower and other crucifers—there's strong evidence of their brain-protective effects.

Helpful: I'm not a veggie lover, so I roast vegetables with olive oil in the oven to make them more appetizing. Whenever possible, I use brain-healthy spices such as rosemary and turmeric.

STEP 3: Guard your sleep. During the day, harmful waste products accumulate in the brain. These wastes, including the amyloid protein that's linked to Alzheimer's, are mainly eliminated at night during deep (stages 3 and 4) sleep.

Scientific evidence: In a long-term Swedish study, men who reported poor sleep were 1.5 times more likely to develop Alzheimer's than those with better sleep.

Regardless of your age, you need a good night's sleep. While ideal sleep times vary depending on the person, sleeping less than six hours or more than nine hours nightly is linked to increased risk for cardiovascular disease—another Alzheimer's risk factor. If you don't feel rested when you wake up, talk to your doctor about your sleep quality.

What I do: I often take a 10-minute nap during the day. Brief naps (especially between 2 pm and 4 pm, which syncs with most people's circadian rhythms) can be restorative.

STEP 4: Don't be a loner. Having regular social interaction is strongly associated with healthy aging.

Scientific evidence: Older adults who frequently spend time with others—for example, sharing meals and volunteering—have about a 70% lower rate of cognitive decline than those who don't socialize much.

What I do: To stay socially active, I regularly Skype, attend conferences and stay in touch with other scientists and postdoc students.

If you're lonely, any form of social interaction is better than none. One study found that people who used computers regularly—to write e-mails, for example—were less lonely than those who didn't. If you can't connect in person, do a video chat or Facebook update at least once a day.

Also helpful: Having a pet. Pets are sometimes better listeners than spouses!

STEP 5: Stay calm. People who are often stressed are more likely to experience brain shrinkage.

Scientific evidence: In a three-year study of people with mild cognitive impairment (a condition that often precedes Alzheimer's), those with severe anxiety had a 135% increased risk for Alzheimer's, compared with those who were calmer.

What I do: I go for long walks.

Other great stress reducers: Having a positive mental attitude, deep breathing, yoga, tai chi, meditation—and even watching funny movies. Practice what works for you.

STEP 6: Push yourself intellectually. So-called "brain workouts" help prevent Alzheimer's—perhaps by increasing cognitive reserve (the stored memories/cognitive skills that you can draw on later in life)…and possibly by accelerating the growth of new brain cells.

Scientific evidence: In an important study, older adults (including those with a genetic risk factor for Alzheimer's) who frequently read, played board games or engaged in other mental activities were able to postpone the development of the disease by almost a decade.

But don't fool yourself—if you're an accomplished pianist, then banging out a tune won't help much even though a nonmusician is likely to benefit from learning to play. Push your mental abilities—do math problems in your head, memorize a poem, become a tutor, etc.

What I do: To challenge myself intellectually, I read novels and practice my foreign language skills—I do research in Latin America, so I work on my Spanish.

Is It Really Alzheimer's? Many People Diagnosed With This Disease Don't Actually Have It

Zaldy S. Tan, MD, MPH, assistant professor of medicine at Harvard Medical School and director of the Preventive Health in Aging Program at Brigham and Women's Hospital, both in Boston. He has been an investigator with the Framingham Heart Study for more than a decade, where his research has focused on Alzheimer's disease and related dementias. He is the author of *Age-Proof Your Mind: Detect, Delay and Prevent Memory Loss—Before It's Too Late.*

Alzheimer's disease is a devastating condition for which there is no effective treatment.

What you may not know: Certain people who think they have Alzheimer's actually may have a condition that is treatable. Unless the misdiagnosis is identified, these people will not only be given ineffective and potentially dangerous treatment, but their real problem also will go untreated. *Conditions that can mimic Alzheimer's…*

DEPRESSION

Cognitive impairments due to depression are known as pseudodementia. Because of a depression-induced lack of attention, which makes it difficult to form and process effective memories, patients may forget appointments or have difficulty remembering names. They also may have trouble concentrating, learning new things and even recognizing faces. This type of dementia, unlike Alzheimer's, is potentially reversible.

Distinguishing signs: Sleep disturbances are more likely to occur with depression than with early-stage Alzheimer's disease. For example, depressed patients may have early morning awakenings or experience difficulty falling asleep at night (typically marked by tossing and turning in bed). They can also have unexplained tearfulness as well as a lack of interest in things that they used to enjoy, a condition called anhedonia.

Treatment: If depression is the culprit, consider talk therapy or an antidepressant, such as *citalopram* (Celexa) or *sertraline* (Zoloft). An antidepressant can usually treat the forgetfulness associated with depression, but it may take several weeks to determine whether a particular drug/dose is going to work. You might also ask your doctor about Saint-John's-wort and other over-the-counter (OTC) natural remedies.

HYPOTHYROIDISM

Thyroid hormone is essential for the growth and maintenance of brain tissue. Patients with low levels of this hormone, a condition known as hypothyroidism, have trouble thinking clearly and can become forgetful or depressed.

Distinguishing signs: A person is diagnosed with hypothyroidism when a blood test shows that his/her thyroid stimulating hormone (TSH) level is above 5.5 mU/L. In addition to memory problems, hypothyroidism also may cause constipation, sudden weight gain and/or dry skin and brittle hair.

Treatment: Most patients can maintain normal thyroid levels, and regain normal mental functions, by taking a once-daily dose of levothyroxine (Synthroid), a thyroid hormone.

MEDICATIONS

Certain prescription and OTC drugs (most commonly, allergy and sleep medicines containing diphenhydramine) can impair memory. These medicines are said to be anti-cholinergic—that is, they decrease the function of the neurotransmitter acetylcholine, which allows brain cells to transfer information and communicate with each other. Multiple drugs may also interact in a way that causes such symptoms.

Distinguishing signs: Memory or behavior changes begin days or weeks after a new medication is started or the drug dose is changed.

Treatment: Avoid OTC medicines that affect memory. In cases such as urinary incontinence or Parkinson's disease, where your doctor needs to prescribe a prescription anticholinergic, ask to start on a low dose to minimize this side effect. Review all medications with your doctor to avoid harmful interactions.

NPH

It's estimated that up to 200,000 older adults in the US have excessive accumulation of fluid on the brain, a condition known as normal pressure hydrocephalus (NPH). The fluid presses on the brain and can cause memory loss and other symptoms that may mimic Alzheimer's.

Distinguishing signs: Most patients with NPH have three main symptoms—an unsteady gait (in the early stages)…followed by urinary incontinence…and cognitive impairments (in later stages). With Alzheimer's, the order is reversed—memory loss and/or other cognitive problems occur first, followed in later stages of the disease by problems with bladder control and gait.

Treatment: NPH can potentially be corrected by inserting a shunt, a tube in the brain that drains excess fluid. However, the surgical procedure is not recommended until after the diagnosis is confirmed by an MRI of the brain and a trial removal of a small amount of fluid through a lumbar tap results in improved memory and/or gait.

NUTRITIONAL DEFICIENCIES

Vitamin B-12. About 10% to 15% of adults age 60 and older have low vitamin B-12 levels. A deficiency of B-12 can damage the my-elin layer that envelops certain nerves, causing memory problems and difficulties with gait and balance.

Distinguishing signs: Besides having trouble walking, patients with a B-12 deficiency may suffer from pins-and-needles sensations, even from a light touch.

Treatment: Severe deficiencies are treated with injections of vitamin B-12. Oral vitamin B-12 can be given to people who are able to absorb sufficient amounts. (In some people, age-related changes to the digestive system prevent proper absorption of this vitamin.) Gait and/or memory may improve as early as a month or two after treatment begins.

•**Thiamine (vitamin B-1).** Heavy alcohol use, anorexia, bariatric surgery and sometimes rapidly growing malignant tumors can cause a severe deficiency of thiamine (vitamin B-1). If this condition becomes chronic, patients may have difficulty walking straight and will also have cognitive problems that can resemble those of Alzheimer's disease. Severe malnutrition also may cause confusion.

Distinguishing signs: Patients may suffer fatigue, loss of mental alertness, depression and abdominal discomfort. Blood tests will show thiamine levels that are close to zero.

Treatment: Severely low thiamine is an emergency in the acute phase. Patients who receive an intravenous thiamine infusion in time, and maintain adequate thiamine levels afterward, may recover and regain their physical/mental abilities. However, those who continue to have low thiamine (often because of chronic alcohol consumption) may suffer permanent cognitive damage.

STROKE

When a person has a series of mini (warning) strokes, it can lead to a type of vascular dementia known as multi-infarct dementia, which can be mistaken for Alzheimer's.

Multi-infarct dementia occurs when damaged blood vessels in the brain slow (but don't completely stop) normal circulation. Reductions in blood and the oxygen it carries can damage brain cells and impair memory and other cognitive abilities—but usually without the motor deficits that accompany a stroke, such as weakness of a limb or slow and/or garbled speech.

Distinguishing signs: Multi-infarct dementia can cause rapid changes in mental functions, sometimes within a few weeks to a month. With Alzheimer's disease, these changes typically occur slowly but steadily over several years.

Treatment: Multi-infarct dementia usually can be diagnosed with a CT or MRI scan showing characteristic changes in the brain. Unfortunately, existing brain damage can't be reversed, although future damage may be avoided. The goal of treatment is to prevent additional vascular damage and cognitive declines by treating the underlying risk factors, such as high blood pressure.

Best Workouts to Keep Your Brain "Buff"

Cynthia R. Green, PhD, a practicing clinical psychologist and the founder and president of Memory Arts, LLC, a brain-health and memory fitness consulting service in Montclair, New Jersey, TotalBrainHealth.com. She is also founding director of the Memory Enhancement Program at the Icahn School of Medicine at Mount Sinai in New York City. She is author of *Your Best Brain Ever: A Complete Guide & Workout.*

We all want to keep our brains in top shape. But are crossword puzzles, online classes and the other such activities that we've been hearing about for years the best ways to do that? Not really.

Now: To improve memory and preserve overall cognitive function, the latest research reveals that it takes more than quiet puzzle-solving and streaming lectures.

Even more intriguing: Some activities that we once thought were time wasters may actually help build intellectual capacity and other cognitive functions.

To learn more about the most effective ways to keep your brain "buff," we talked to Dr. Cynthia R. Green, a psychologist and a leading brain trainer.

A HEALTHY BRAIN

The most important steps to keep your brain performing at optimal levels are lifestyle choices…

• **Getting aerobic exercise** (at least 150 minutes per week).

• **Maintaining a healthy body weight.**

• **Not smoking.**

• **Eating a diet that emphasizes fruits and vegetables and is low in refined sugar and white flour**—two of the biggest dietary threats to brain health that have recently been identified by researchers.

Additional benefits are possible with regular brain workouts. In the past, experts thought that nearly any game or activity that challenges you to think would improve your general brain functioning.

What research now tells us: An increasing body of evidence shows that improved memory requires something more—you need to work against a clock. Games with a time limit force you to think quickly and with agility. These are the factors that lead to improved memory and mental focus. *Among Dr. Green's favorite brain workouts—aim for at least 30 minutes daily of any combination of the activities below…*

BRAINY COMPUTER GAMES

Specialized brain-training computer programs (such as Lumosity, Fit Brains and CogniFit) are no longer the darlings of the health community. Formerly marketed as a fun way to reduce one's risk for dementia, recent evidence has not supported that claim.

These programs do provide, however, a variety of activities that may help improve intellectual performance, attention, memory and mental flexibility. Lumosity and other programs are a good option for people who enjoy a regimented brain workout, including such activities as remembering sequences and ignoring distractions. Monthly prices range from $4.99 to $19.95.

Other options to consider trying…

• **Action video games.** These games were once considered "brain-numbing" activities that kept players from developing intellectual and social skills. Recent research, however, shows that action video games can promote mental focus, flexible thinking, and decision-making and problem-solving skills. Because these games are timed, they also require quick responses from the players.

Good choices: World of Warcraft, The Elder Scrolls and Guild Wars, all of which involve role-playing by assuming the identity of various characters to battle foes and complete quests, often with other virtual players. These games are available in DVD format for Mac or PC and with an online subscription for virtual play.

Caveat: An hour or two can be a brain booster, but don't overdo it. Too much role-playing takes you away from real-life interactions.

• **Free brain-boosting computer game for a cause.** At *FreeRice.com*, you can answer fun and challenging questions in such subjects as English vocabulary, foreign languages, math and humanities. With each correct answer, the United Nations World Food Programme donates 10 grains of rice to a Third World country. To date, players have "earned" a total of nearly 100 billion grains of rice—enough to create more than 10 million meals.

To increase the challenge: Set a timer so that you must work against the clock.

APPS FOR YOUR BRAIN

If you'd prefer to use an "app"—a software application that you can use on a smartphone or similar electronic device—there are several good options. *Among the best fun/challenging apps (free on Android and Apple)…*

• **Words with Friends.** This ever-popular game allows you to play a Scrabble-like game against your friends who have also downloaded the app on an electronic device. The game provides even more benefits if it's used with the time-clock feature.

• **Word Streak with Friends (formerly Scramble with Friends) is a timed find-a-word game.** You can play on your own or with friends.

• **Elevate was named Apple's Best App of 2014.** It provides a structured game environment that feels more like a test, focusing on reading, writing and math skills, than a game. Still, this timed app will give Apple users a good brain challenge.

TECH-FREE OPTIONS

If you'd rather not stare at the screen of a computer or some other electronic device for your brain workout, here are some good options…

• **Tech-free games.** SET is a fast-paced card game that tests your visual perception skills. Players race to find a set of three matching cards (based on color, shape, number or shading) from an array of cards placed on a table.

Bonus: This game can be played by one player or as many people as can fit around the table. The winner of dozens of "Best Game" awards, including the high-IQ group Mensa's Select award, SET is fun for kids and adults alike.

Another good choice: Boggle, which challenges you to create words from a given set of letter cubes within a three-minute period. It can be played by two or more people.

• **Drumming.** Playing any musical instrument requires attention and a keen sense of timing. Basic drumming is a great activity for beginner musicians (especially if you don't have the finger dexterity for piano or guitar).

Even better: Join a drumming circle, which provides the extra challenge of matching your timing and rhythm to the rest of the drummers, along with opportunities for socialization.

Bonus: Research has demonstrated that some forms, such as African djembe drumming, count as a low- to moderate-intensity activity that may reduce blood pressure, which helps protect the brain from blood vessel damage.

• **Meditation.** This practice improves cognitive function and sensory processing and promotes mental focus. Meditating for about 30 minutes daily has also been linked to greater blood flow to the brain and increased gray matter (associated with positive emotions, memory and decision-making). The benefits have even been seen among some people with early-stage neurodegenerative diseases, such as Alzheimer's disease.

A good way to get started: Begin with a simple "mindful eating" exercise—spend the first five minutes of each meal really focusing on what you're eating. Don't talk, read the paper or watch TV…just savor the food. Eventually, you'll want to expand this level of attention to other parts of your day. Such mindfulness habits are a good complement to a regular meditation practice.

•**Coloring.** If you have kids or grandkids, don't just send them off with their crayons. Color with them.

Even better: Get one of the new breed of coloring books with complex designs for adults. While there hasn't been specific research addressing the brain benefits of coloring, this form of play has been shown to reduce stress in children, and it is thought to boost creativity and have a meditative quality. You can find coloring books made for adults at bookstores and art-supply stores (or see pages 117–120 for samples).

For a Sharper Brain, Eat These 4 Foods

Drew Ramsey, MD, an assistant clinical professor of psychiatry at Columbia University College of Physicians and Surgeons in New York City. Dr. Ramsey is also coauthor of *The Happiness Diet: A Nutritional Prescription for a Sharp Brain, Balanced Mood, and Lean, Energized Body* and *Fifty Shades of Kale: 50 Fresh and Satisfying Recipes That Are Bound to Please.*

We all know that a strong cup of coffee can give us that extra mental boost we may need to complete a brain-draining project or meet a tight deadline.

What works even better: Strategic eating is a healthful and reliable way to improve your ability to concentrate for the long haul—not just for a few hours at a time when you're hyped-up on caffeine.

There's no single food that will suddenly have you speed-reading a book in one sitting, but you can improve your overall powers of concentration by including the following foods in your diet…

•**Eggs.** When it comes to mental focus, it doesn't get much better than eggs! They're a leading source of a nutrient called choline, a precursor to the neurotransmitter acetylcholine—a key molecule of learning.

Eggs (including the yolks) also contain a variety of B vitamins, most of which have been stripped from the refined carbs that are so ubiquitous in the typical American diet. In particular, eggs are rich in vitamins B-6 and B-12, which are crucial for carrying out most cognitive functions (three large eggs will give you about half of your daily B-12 requirement)… and vitamin B-9 (also known as folate).

For optimal brain health, include up to 12 eggs in your diet each week. While cholesterol in one's diet has only a minimal effect on blood levels of cholesterol, consult your doctor for advice on appropriate intake of eggs if cholesterol is a concern.

•**Mussels.** Three ounces of mussels—which is a modest serving—contain 20 micrograms (mcg) of vitamin B-12 (that's nearly 10 times your daily requirement). Even a mild deficiency of this crucial brain-boosting vitamin can impair concentration and lead to fuzzy thinking.

But that's not all. Three ounces of mussels will also give you 430 mg of docosahexaenoic acid (DHA)—the equivalent of two to three typical fish oil supplement capsules. DHA is a type of omega-3 fatty acid needed for healthy brain function. Mussels are also loaded with zinc, a nutritional workhorse involved in more than 100 chemical reactions in the brain. Enjoy mussels twice a month.

Don't like mussels? Other smart brain-boosting seafood selections include oysters (six oysters deliver three to four times your daily zinc needs)…anchovies, which have more omega-3s than tuna…and clams, which are an excellent source of vitamin B-12.

Tasty choices: Caesar salad with anchovies…clam chowder…or pasta alle vongole (with clams).

•**Beef.** You've probably heard that eating too much red meat is linked to heart disease and even some types of cancer. However, you can minimize these risks and maximize your brain-power with a few small servings per week.

Here's why: Beef is a potent source of heme iron (the most absorbable form), which is needed to transport oxygen through the blood and to the brain.

What I recommend: Opt for grass-fed beef. It has fewer calories, less fat and more nutrients (such as vitamin E) than conventional beef. Meat from grass-fed animals has two to three times more conjugated linoleic acid (CLA) than meat from grain-fed animals. CLA helps protect the brain by counteracting the effects of harmful stress hormones.

Try to have grass-fed beef once or twice a week—but give it a supporting role instead of making it the star of your meal. Think grass-fed vegetable beef stew instead of a large steak.

Note: Even though grass-fed beef is more expensive than conventional beef, you can save by opting for nontraditional cuts, such as beef shank, stew meats and roasts. If you are a vegetarian or vegan, black beans are an excellent substitute.

• **Cruciferous vegetables.** Take your pick—the list includes brussels sprouts, kale, arugula, bok choy, cauliflower and collard greens. As members of the Brassica plant family, these veggies contain sulfur-based anti-inflammatory compounds that help protect the brain. One of these compounds, sulforaphane, has even been shown to improve memory and learning after brain injury.

Aim for at least two cups of cruciferous vegetables daily—I put that much in my kale-blueberry smoothie every morning!

Note: Consult your doctor before changing the amount of leafy greens you eat if you take *warfarin*, a blood thinner, since vitamin K–rich foods may interact.

Other good choices: Add purple cabbage to a stir-fry...or mash cauliflower instead of potatoes and season with brain-boosting turmeric and black pepper (to increase the absorption of turmeric).

4 Supplements That Can Impair Your Brain

Cynthia Kuhn, PhD, professor of pharmacology, cancer biology, psychiatry and behavioral sciences at Duke University School of Medicine. Dr. Kuhn is also coauthor, with Scott Swartzwelder, PhD, and Wilkie Wilson, PhD, of *Buzzed: The Straight Facts About the Most Used and Abused Drugs from Alcohol to Ecstas*y.

I t's hardly news that supplements—just like drugs—can have physical side effects.

Recent development: Researchers are now learning more and more about unwanted mental changes that can occur when taking popular supplements (such as herbs and hormones).

These supplements can be a hidden cause of depression, anxiety, mania and other mental changes because patients—and their doctors—often don't realize how these products can affect the brain.

Supplements that may cause unwanted mental changes...

MELATONIN

Melatonin is among the most popular supplements for treating insomnia, jet lag and other sleep disorders. Melatonin is a natural hormone that's released by the pineal gland at night and readily enters the brain. Unlike many sleep aids, it doesn't render you unconscious or put you to sleep—it causes subtle brain changes that make you "ready" for sleep.

Studies have shown that people who take melatonin in the late afternoon or early evening tend to fall asleep more quickly when they go to bed. The amount of melatonin used in scientific studies ranges from 0.1 mg to 0.5 mg. However, the products in health-food stores typically contain much higher doses—usually 1 mg to 5 mg. Supplemental melatonin also may become less effective over time, which encourages people to increase the doses even more.

Effects on the brain: In people with depression, melatonin may improve sleep, but it may worsen their depression symptoms, according to the National Institutes of Health.

What to do: Melatonin can help when used short term for such problems as jet lag. It is not particularly effective as a long-term solution for other causes of insomnia.

ST. JOHN'S WORT

St. John's wort is probably the most studied herb for treating depression. Researchers who analyzed data from 29 international studies recently concluded that St. John's wort was as effective as prescription antidepressants for treating minor to moderate depression.

St. John's wort appears to be safe, particularly when it's used under the supervision of a physician. However, it can cause unwanted mental changes.

Effects on the brain: St. John's wort may increase brain levels of "feel good" neurotransmitters, including serotonin and dopamine. But unwanted mental changes that may occur in anyone taking St. John's wort include anxiety, irritability and vivid dreams. It may also lead to mania (a condition characterized by periods of overactivity, excessive excitement and lack of inhibitions)—especially in individuals who are also using antipsychotic drugs.

Caution: This supplement should never be combined with a prescription selective serotonin reuptake inhibitor (SSRI) antidepressant, such as *sertraline* (Zoloft) or *paroxetine* (Paxil). Taking St. John's wort with an SSRI can cause serotonin syndrome, excessive brain levels of serotonin that can increase body temperature, heart rate and blood pressure—conditions that are all potentially fatal. It also can interact with certain drugs such as oral contraceptives and immunosuppressant medications.

What to do: If you have depression, do not self-medicate with St. John's wort. Always talk to your doctor first if you are interested in trying this supplement.

TESTOSTERONE

Older men whose testosterone levels are declining (as is normal with aging) are often tempted to get a prescription for supplemental "T," which is advertised (but not proven) to improve their ability to get erections. Some women also use testosterone patches or gels (in much lower doses than men) to increase sexual desire and arousal.

Effects on the brain: If your testosterone is low, taking supplemental doses may cause a pleasant—but slight—increase in energy. However, with very high doses, such as those taken by bodybuilders, side effects may include aggression and mood swings. Men and women may experience withdrawal symptoms—such as depression and loss of appetite—when they stop taking it.

Testosterone replacement for men is FDA approved only for those with a clinical deficiency—defined as blood levels under 300 nanograms per deciliter (ng/dL).

What to do: Testosterone has been shown to increase sexual desire in women—it is not FDA approved for women but may be prescribed "off-label." The evidence supporting testosterone's ability to improve sexual function and well-being in normally aging men is weaker—unless they have been proven on more than one occasion to have low testosterone and related symptoms. Both men and women should take testosterone only under the supervision of a doctor.

WEIGHT-LOSS SUPPLEMENTS

Two ingredients that are commonly used in weight-loss supplements, beta-phenylethylamine (PEA) and P-synephrine, are said to increase energy and metabolism and burn extra calories.

Effects on the brain: Both PEA and P-synephrine (a compound found in supplements made from bitter orange) can make you feel jittery and anxious, particularly when they are combined with stimulants such as caffeine.

Many weight-loss and "energy" products are complicated cocktails of active ingredients that haven't been adequately studied—nor have they been approved by the FDA. They're risky because they've been linked to dangerous increases in blood pressure.

Important: There is little evidence that any of these products is particularly effective as a weight-loss aid.

59

What to do: Don't rely on weight-loss supplements. To lose weight, you need to decrease your food intake and increase your exercise levels—no supplement can accomplish that!

Want to Boost Short-Term Memory? Watch a Funny Video

Gurinder Singh Bains, MD, PhD, assistant professor and primary research coordinator, Loma Linda University School of Allied Health Professions, Loma Linda, California. His study was published in *Alternative Therapies*.

You forget that thing that someone told you…this morning. You misplace your keys. You walk into the kitchen to do something…but once you get there, you forget what it is.

What you're experiencing is a decline in short-term memory. It starts to go down as early as your 40s…and it's perfectly normal. (Forgetting where you live or what your keys are for, that's a different story.)

But wouldn't it be great if there were something simple and easy that you could do to improve it?

There is. In fact it's so simple, it's funny.

HOW RED SKELTON ENHANCES BRAIN POWER

Watching a humorous video for 20 minutes may be all it takes to improve your ability to remember things you've just heard or read, found researchers at Loma Linda University in California. They showed 20 older men and women (average age 70) either a video of Red Skelton (the former clown who had a popular TV comedy show in the 1950s, '60s and early '70s)…or a montage from America's Funniest Home Videos.

None of the participants had any cognitive impairment. However, half of them (10) had diabetes, which is known to contribute to short-term memory loss. An additional 10 participants, who did not have diabetes nor cognitive impairment and were of the same age, were the control group. They did not watch the videos but instead were asked to sit silently in a quiet room.

Before and after watching funny videos…or sitting in silence…the participants took three components of a short-term-memory test. First, a researcher read aloud 15 words, and participants were then asked to say from memory as many as they could remember…a test of learning. The test was repeated five times. The same test was then given with a different list, and then participants were asked to remember what had been on the first list…a test of recall. Finally, participants were given a piece of paper with 50 words on it and asked to circle words that had been on the first list…a test of visual recognition. Finally, a little saliva was swabbed at five different points, including before and after—you'll see why in a moment.

Result? Laughter worked. After watching the humorous videos, the healthy adults did 39% better on the learning test, 44% better on the recall test and 13% better on the visual recognition test. Those with diabetes also saw significant improvements—a 33% boost in learning, a 48% jump in recall and a 17% gain in visual recognition. Sitting silently also seemed to benefit the control group but not nearly as much. Their gains were 24%, 20% and 8%, respectively.

How can a little mirth improve memory? That's where the saliva comes in.

THE STRESS CONNECTION

Saliva contains cortisol, a stress hormone. All of the participants who watched the funny videos experienced a significant decrease in salivary cortisol levels. Stress, as the researchers already knew, suppresses the function of the brain's hippocampus, where short-term memory is pulled together. (Over time, chronic stress can even damage…and shrink…the hippocampus.) Feeling less stress and producing fewer stress hormones, the researchers speculate, is what led to better learning and memory in the video watchers.

This wonderfully simple experiment suggests a wonderfully simple way that we could all boost our short-term memory—watch humorous videos. *There are literally thousands that are easily found online…but here are three good (and free) ones…*

•**The hilarious well-known scene from the *I Love Lucy* TV show**—when Lucy and Ethel get jobs at a candy factory.

•**Comedienne Carol Burnett's spoof on *Gone With the Wind*.**

•**Frasier,** from the TV comedy series *Frasier*, sings "Buttons and Bows."

If you want to stretch out the experience, try these funny full-length movies—*Blazing Saddles* (1974), *Airplane!* (1980), *Raising Arizona* (1987), *A Fish Called Wanda* (1988), *Liar Liar* (1997), *There's Something About Mary* (1998), *Little Miss Sunshine* (2006), *Death at a Funeral* (2007) *and Bridesmaids* (2011).

Of course, you don't have to watch a video to relax and laugh. Although it wasn't studied, it's a reasonable speculation that anything that lowers stress levels may enhance short-term memory. While this is the first research to show memory improvement, other research has shown that humor and laughter stimulate the immune system, make pain more tolerable, improve mood and even reduce markers of inflammation. That's fun with benefits.

Stop Memory Loss

Pamela Wartian Smith, MD, MPH, codirector of the master's program in medical sciences with a concentration in metabolic and nutritional medicine at Morsani College of Medicine at University of South Florida and owner and director of the Michigan-based Center for Personalized Medicine. She is author of *What You Must Know About Memory Loss & How You Can Stop It: A Guide to Proven Techniques and Supplements to Maintain, Strengthen, or Regain Memory.* CFHLL.com

Do you have trouble remembering names and phone numbers? How about where you put things? Do you sometimes struggle to come up with the right word?

Mild forgetfulness, known as age-related memory impairment, is a natural part of getting older. By age 75, a person's memory has declined, on average, by about 43%. After age 75, the hippocampus, the part of the brain most closely associated with memory, will eventually atrophy at the rate of 1% to 2% each year.

But you can improve memory with over-the-counter supplements—if you choose the right ones. Here are the supplements I find most effective with my patients. You can take several of these if you choose. You could start with phosphatidylserine and add others depending on your personal needs. For example, if you're taking a medication that depletes CoQ10, you might want to take that supplement. Or if you're under stress, add ashwagandha root. Of course, always check with your doctor before starting any new supplement. To find a practitioner trained in this field, go to *Metabolic-Anti-AgingSpecialist.com.*

•**Phosphatidylserine (PS).** Most people haven't heard of it, but PS is one of my first choices for mild memory loss. It's a naturally occurring phospholipid (a molecule that contains two fatty acids) that increases the body's production of acetylcholine and other neurotransmitters. It improves cell-to-cell communication and "nourishes" the brain by improving glucose metabolism.

Studies have shown that healthy people who take PS are more likely to maintain their ability to remember things. For those who have already experienced age-related memory loss, PS can improve memory. It's also thought to improve symptoms caused by some forms of dementia.

Typical dose: 300 mg daily. You're unlikely to notice any side effects.

•**Co-enzyme Q10 (CoQ10).** This is another naturally occurring substance found in many foods (such as fatty fish, meats, nuts, fruits and vegetables) and in nearly all of your body's tissues. CoQ10 increases the production of adenosine triphosphate, a molecule that enhances energy production within cells. It's also a potent antioxidant that reduces cell-damaging inflammation in the brain and other parts of the body.

People with degenerative brain disorders, such as Alzheimer's, tend to have lower levels of CoQ10. Studies suggest that supplemental CoQ10 improves memory by protecting brain cells from oxidative damage.

Important: If you're taking a medication that depletes CoQ10—examples include statins

61

(for lowering cholesterol)…metformin (for diabetes)…and beta-blockers (for heart disease and other conditions)—you'll definitely want to take a supplement. I often recommend it for people age 50 and older because the body's production of CoQ10 declines with age. Hard exercise also depletes it.

Typical dose: Between 30 mg and 360 mg daily. Ask your health-care professional how much you need—it will depend on medication use and other factors. Side effects are rare but may include insomnia, agitation and digestive problems such as diarrhea and heartburn.

●**Acetyl-L-carnitine.** A study that looked at people with mild cognitive impairment (an intermediate stage between age-related memory impairment and dementia) found that acetyl-L-carnitine improved memory, attention and even verbal fluency.

Acetyl-L-carnitine (it is derived from an amino acid) is a versatile molecule. It's used by the body to produce acetyl-choline, the main neurotransmitter involved in memory. It slows the rate of neurotransmitter decay, increases oxygen availability and helps convert body fat into energy.

Typical dose: 1,000 mg to 2,000 mg daily. Check with your health-care professional before starting acetyl-L-carnitine to see what dose is best for you. If your kidneys are not functioning perfectly, you may need a lower dose. Some people may notice a slight fishy body odor. In my experience, you can prevent this by taking 50 mg to 100 mg of vitamin B-2 at the same time you take acetyl-L-carnitine.

●**Ashwagandha root.** This is an herb that improves the repair and regeneration of brain cells (neurons) and inhibits the body's production of acetylcholinesterase, an enzyme that degrades acetylcholine. It also improves the ability to deal with both physical and emotional stress—both of which have been linked to impaired memory and cognitive decline.

Typical dose: 500 mg to 2,000 mg daily. Start with the lower dose. If after a month you don't notice that your memory and focus have improved, take a little more. GI disturbances are possible but not common.

Warning: Don't take this supplement if you're also taking a prescription medication that has cholinesterase-inhibiting effects, such as *donepezil* (Aricept) or *galantamine* (Razadyne). Ask your health-care professional whether any of your medications have this effect.

●**Ginkgo biloba.** Among the most studied herbal supplements, ginkgo is an antioxidant that protects the hippocampus from age-related atrophy. It's a vaso-dilator that helps prevent blood clots, improves brain circulation and reduces the risk for vascular dementia, a type of dementia associated with impaired blood flow to the brain. It also increases the effects of serotonin, a neurotransmitter that's involved in mood and learning.

Bonus: In animal studies, ginkgo appears to block the formation of amyloid, the protein that has been linked to Alzheimer's disease. There's strong evidence that ginkgo can stabilize and possibly improve memory.

Typical dose: 60 mg to 120 mg daily. Most people won't have side effects, but ginkgo is a blood thinner that can react with other anticoagulants. If you're taking warfarin or another blood thinner (including aspirin and fish oil), be sure to check with your health-care professional before taking ginkgo.

●**Fish oil.** Much of the brain consists of DHA (docosahexaenoic acid), one of the main omega-3 fatty acids. It is essential for brain health. People who take fish-oil supplements have improved brain circulation and a faster transmission of nerve signals.

Studies have found that people who eat a lot of fatty fish have a lower risk for mild cognitive impairment than people who tend to eat little or no fatty fish. One study found that people with age-related memory impairment achieved better scores on memory tests when they took daily DHA supplements.

Typical dose: 2,000 mg daily if you're age 50 or older. Look for a combination supplement that includes equal amounts of DHA and EPA (another omega-3). Fish-oil supplements can increase the effects of blood-thinning medications such as aspirin and warfarin if the dose is above 3,000 mg a day.

•**Huperzine A.** Extracted from a Chinese moss, this is a cholinesterase inhibitor that increases brain levels of acetylcholine. It also protects brain cells from too-high levels of glutamate, another neurotransmitter.

Huperzine A may improve memory and could even help delay symptoms of Alzheimer's disease. A study conducted by the National Institute of Aging found that patients with mild-to-moderate Alzheimer's who took huperzine A had improvements in cognitive functions.

Recommended dose: 400 mcg daily. Don't take it if you're already taking a prescription cholinesterase inhibitor (as discussed in the "Ashwagandha root" section).

Alzheimer's Symptoms Reversed!

Dale Bredesen, MD, the Augustus Rose Professor of Neurology and director of the Mary S. Easton Center for Alzheimer's Disease Research, the Alzheimer's Disease Program and Neurodegenerative Disease Research in the David Geffen School of Medicine, UCLA. He is founding president of the Buck Institute for Research on Aging in Novato, California.

Can Alzheimer's symptoms be reversed? A breakthrough treatment suggests that they can. In a study recently published in the journal *Aging,* Dale Bredesen, MD, director of the Alzheimer's Disease Program at UCLA's David Geffen School of Medicine, presented an all-natural, multicomponent treatment program that reversed memory loss in four people with Alzheimer's and in five people with either subjective cognitive impairment or mild cognitive impairment (the stages of memory loss that typically precede Alzheimer's).

We interviewed Dr. Bredesen, who explained that his program is based on a new theory about why people get Alzheimer's. *This theory was developed over two decades of cellular and animal research at the Buck Institute for Research on Aging and UCLA...*

NEW THINKING

The current, widely accepted theory of Alzheimer's says that the protein beta-amyloid forms plaques outside neurons in the brain...somehow triggering the production of abnormal tau tangles inside neurons...thereby interfering with synapses, the information-laden connections between neurons that create memory and other mental activity.

New thinking: Normal mental function depends on a balance between synaptoblastic (synapse-making) and synaptoclastic (synapse-destroying) activity. If there is more synaptoclastic activity, memory loss may ensue. If there is chronic synaptoclastic activity, our research suggests that Alzheimer's occurs.

My colleagues and I have identified 36 unique synapse-affecting factors (including beta-amyloid). Addressing only one or two of these factors—with a drug, for example—will not reverse Alzheimer's. But addressing many factors—10, 20 or more—can effectively reverse the symptoms.

Here are several key factors in what we call the MEND (Metabolic Enhancement for NeuroDegeneration) program—factors anyone can use to prevent, slow, stop or potentially even reverse memory loss...

RESTORING MEMORY

Synapse-making and synapse-destroying factors function in a "loop" that develops momentum, like a snowball rolling downhill. In the synapse-destroying momentum of Alzheimer's, you gradually lose memories, ultimately even basic ones such as the faces of loved ones. But because the synapse-making factors in the MEND program are so effective, they can reverse the momentum of Alzheimer's. The more of them that you incorporate into your daily life, the more momentum there is to protect and restore memory.

•**Optimize diet.** Eliminate simple carbohydrates such as anything made from white flour and/or refined sugar. Don't eat processed foods with either "trans fats" or "partially hydrogenated vegetable oil" on the label. If you're sensitive to gluten, minimize your consumption of gluten-containing foods, such as wheat and rye (there are simple tests to determine whether you are indeed gluten-sensitive). Emphasize fruits and vegetables. Eat nonfarmed fish for neuron-protecting omega-3 fatty acids.

Why it works: This dietary approach reduces inflammation and high levels of insulin (the hormone that regulates blood sugar), both of which are synapse-destroying.

Important: Dietary changes have more impact than any other factor in preventing or reversing memory loss.

Helpful: Four books that have diets consistent with MEND are *Eat to Live* by Joel Furhman, MD...*The Blood Sugar Solution* by Mark Hyman, MD...*The Spectrum* by Dean Ornish, MD...and *Grain Brain* by David Perlmutter, MD.

• **Have a nightly "fast."** Don't eat three hours before bedtime. Ideally, 12 hours should pass between the last time you eat at night and when you eat breakfast.

Example: Dinner ending at 8:00 pm and breakfast starting at 8:00 am.

Why it works: This eating pattern enhances autophagy (the body's ability to "clean up" dysfunctional cells, such as beta-amyloid) and ketosis (the generation of ketones, molecules that can help protect neurons). It also reduces insulin.

• **Reduce stress.** Pick a relaxing, enjoyable activity—walking in the woods, yoga, meditation, playing the piano, etc.—and do it once a day or every other day for at least 20 to 30 minutes.

Why it works: Stress destroys neurons in the hippocampus, the part of the brain that helps create short- and long-term memory. Stress also boosts cortisol, a synapse-damaging hormone. And stress increases corticotropin-releasing factor (CRF), a hormone linked to Alzheimer's.

• **Optimize sleep.** Sleep seven to eight hours every night.

Why it works: Anatomical changes during sleep flush the brain of toxic, synapse-damaging compounds. If you have trouble sleeping, we have found that 0.5 mg of melatonin at bedtime is the best dose for restorative sleep.

• **Exercise regularly.** I recommend 30 to 60 minutes per day, four to six days per week. Combining aerobic exercise (such as brisk walking) with weight-training is ideal.

Why it works: Among its many benefits, exercise produces brain-derived neurotrophic factor (BDNF), a powerfully synaptoblastic compound.

• **Stimulate your brain.** Brain-training exercises and games stimulate and improve your ability to remember, pay attention, process information quickly and creatively navigate daily life.

Why it works: Just as using muscle builds muscle, using synapses builds synapses. (Scientists call this ability of the brain to change and grow plasticity.)

• **Take folate, vitamin B-6 and vitamin B-12.** These three nutrients can reduce blood levels of the amino acid homocysteine, which is linked to an increase in tau, increased age-related shrinkage of the hippocampus and double the risk for Alzheimer's disease.

However: To work, these supplements must undergo a biochemical process called methylation—and many older people don't "methylate" well, rendering the supplements nearly useless. To avoid the problem, take a form of the supplements that already is methylated (or activated)—folate as L-methylfolate, B-6 as pyridoxal-5-phosphate and B-12 as methylcobalamin.

• **Take other targeted supplements.** Along with the three B vitamins, there are many other supplements that target synaptoblastic and synaptoclastic factors. Check with your doctor about the right dosages. The supplements include vitamin D-3 (low levels double the risk for Alzheimer's)...vitamin K-2...vitamin E (as mixed tocopherols and tocotrienols)...the minerals selenium, magnesium and zinc (zinc, for example, lowers copper, which is linked to Alzheimer's)...DHA and EPA (anti-inflammatory omega-3 fatty acids)...coenzyme Q10, N-acetylcysteine, alpha-lipoic acid (they nourish mitochondria, energy-generating structures within cells)...and probiotics (they improve the microbiome, helping to strengthen the lining of the gut, reducing body-wide inflammation).

Also, certain herbs can be helpful. These include curcumin (1 gram per day), ashwagandha (500 mg once or twice per day) and bacopa monnieri (200 mg to 300 mg per day). These have multiple effects, such as reducing inflammation and amyloid-beta peptide and enhancing neurotransmission.

Many Food Cans Still Contain BPA

The chemical bisphenol A often is used to line the inside of metal food cans to prevent food from touching the metal. It has been linked to health problems that affect the brain and the nervous system. While used less often than in the past, BPA still appears in about one-third of cans studied. Manufacturers are not required to identify cans with or without BPA. Among brands found to be BPA-free are Amy's, Earth's Best Organic, Health Valley, Seneca, Sprouts Farmers Market and Tyson. For more information on brands using BPA and those that are BPA-free, go to *EWG.org/re search/bpa-canned-food*.

Study of 252 brands made by 119 companies between January and August 2014 by researchers at Environmental Working Group, an advocacy organization in Washington, DC.

Sleep and Alzheimer's

A long-term study of initially healthy 65-year-olds found that those who slept the least (about five hours or less without waking) tended to have fewer neurons (brain cells) in a part of the brain that controls sleep.

Also: Many in the study who developed Alzheimer's disease were those who had fewer neurons and less sleep.

To protect your brain: Keep neurons healthy with good sleep habits, and seek treatment if you suspect you may have a sleep disorder.

Andrew Lim, MD, assistant professor of neurology, University of Toronto, Canada.

Next Steps If You Suspect Early-Onset Alzheimer's Disease

Susan M. Maixner, MD, clinical associate professor of psychiatry, director of the Geropsychiatry Program, director of the geriatric psychiatry clinic at the University of Michigan Health System, and psychiatric consultant at Arbor Hospice, Ann Arbor.

If you haven't seen the acclaimed movie *Still Alice*, starring Julianne Moore, who won an Academy Award for her performance, all we can say, without being "spoilers," is that the movie provides powerful food for thought for anyone concerned that dementia is setting in—and happening way too soon. The movie is about a linguistics professor and mother of three who is diagnosed with Alzheimer's disease at the tender age of 50.

For those of you who are middle-aged and feeling more distracted and forgetful—or more easily agitated than you once were—the movie will shake you up. It's not always easy to tell whether these symptoms are simply due to stress and multitasking or the beginnings of true cognitive decline. So how can you tell?

SUSPICIOUS SIGNS

The key symptom to look out for is trouble managing "bills and pills," said Susan Maixner, MD, a clinical associate professor of psychiatry and director of the Geropsychiatry Program at the University of Michigan Health System. If you are younger than 65 and bill-paying becomes increasingly difficult to keep track of and if you find yourself forgetting to take medications or doubling up on doses (a danger in and of itself), you may be in the danger zone for early-onset Alzheimer's disease. For those still working, being unable to retain information for work, such as frequently used computer passwords, may be a very early sign of cognitive difficulties, said Dr. Maixner.

A decline in short-term memory, such as too often forgetting whether or not you paid that bill or took that med, usually comes first when early-onset Alzheimer's sets in, said Dr. Maixner. Other telltale signs are the same as those for Alzheimer's in older age groups—get-

65

ting lost while driving, repeating yourself, inability to plan or to solve problems, confusion with time or place, the inability to comprehend visual images (for example, not recognizing acquaintances), difficulty writing or speaking, often misplacing things, failing judgment, social withdrawal and change in mood or personality, such as feeling more short-tempered or frustrated.

GETTING DIAGNOSED

The first step to getting a diagnosis is scheduling a thorough medical exam that your family doctor can perform, said Dr. Maixner. "Make sure that you tell your primary care doctor, up front, that you are scheduling the physical exam because you are experiencing memory problems and are concerned about early-onset Alzheimer's," said Dr. Maixner. The exam will be tailored to rule out physical as well as psychological ailments that may be causing the cognitive decline. And, because approximately 20% of early-onset Alzheimer's disease is inherited (genetic), tell your family doctor if you have a family history of dementia. Many primary care physicians won't think to ask this question—so be sure to bring it up, said Dr. Maixner.

Make sure blood work is done to rule out thyroid problems or vitamin deficiencies that can cause memory issues, advised Dr. Maixner. Medications and the use of drugs and alcohol also should be considered. The primary care doctor should then perform in-office cognitive tests, such as the Mini-Mental State Exam or Montreal Cognitive Assessment, which evaluate mental sharpness and short- and long-term memory. If the test results reveal signs of cognitive decline, your doctor should refer you to a geriatric psychiatrist or a neurologist with expertise in managing cognitive disorders such as dementia. The specialist may order an MRI or a CT scan of the brain to rule out whether a stroke, brain injury lesion or tumor may be causing the symptoms. A geriatric psychiatrist also has special training in differentiating dementia from depression, anxiety and other conditions that can accompany memory problems, said Dr. Maixner.

COPING WITH EARLY-ONSET ALZHEIMER'S

So far, there is no cure for Alzheimer's disease. Although progressive worsening of the disease is inevitable, the clock can be turned back on symptoms with lifestyle interventions and medications. It is crucial to keep up physical activity, social interactions and mental stimulation, according to Dr. Maixner. Also, routines, predictability and structure are essential coping tools that will help you or a loved one with early-onset Alzheimer's function better.

Planning about who will manage financial affairs and health decisions is important because if it is Alzheimer's, a time will come when you or your loved one will no longer be able to make those decisions, said Dr. Maixner. Support groups and a 24/7 information hotline that can help with finding a dementia specialist, coping, staying active and legal issues are available through the Alzheimer's Association.

The New "Brain Food"

Want your brain to be as sharp as someone's a decade younger? Eat more spinach and kale. A 10-year study of more than 950 older adults found that those who ate just one or two servings of leafy greens per day had the cognitive abilities of people 11 years younger.

Why it works: The lutein and vitamin K in the greens protect cognitive function.

Important: If you take the blood thinner warfarin, work with your doctor to modify your dosage if you increase your intake of leafy greens.

Martha Clare Morris, ScD, director of nutrition and nutritional epidemiology, Rush University, Chicago.

5

The New Super Foods For Super Health

Foods That Fight Pain—Some Work Even Better Than Drugs

Many of us turn to medications to relieve pain. But research has shown that you can help reduce specific types of pain—and avoid the side effects of drugs—just by choosing the right foods. Here, the common causes of pain and the foods that can help. *Unless otherwise noted, aim to eat the recommended foods daily…*

OSTEOARTHRITIS

Osteoarthritis causes pain and inflammation in the joints.

Best foods: Bing cherries, ginger, avocado oil and soybean oil.

A study in *The Journal of Nutrition* found that men and women who supplemented their diets with Bing cherries (about two cups of cherries throughout the day) had an 18% to 25% drop in C-reactive protein, a sign of inflammation. Bing cherries contain flavonoids, plant-based compounds with antioxidant properties that lower inflammation.

Ginger also contains potent anti-inflammatory agents that can reduce joint pain. A double-blind, placebo-controlled study found that 63% of people who consumed ginger daily had less knee pain when walking or standing. I recommend one to two teaspoons of ground fresh ginger every day.

Avocado oil and soybean oil contain avocado soybean unsaponifiables (ASUs), which reduce inflammation and cartilage damage in arthritis patients.

RHEUMATOID ARTHRITIS

This autoimmune disease causes systemic inflammation—your joints, your heart and even your lungs may be affected.

David Grotto, RD, founder and president of Nutrition Housecall, LLC, a consulting firm based in Chicago that provides nutrition communications, lecturing and consulting services as well as personalized, at-home dietary services. He is author of *The Best Things You Can Eat: For Everything from Aches to Zzzz*. DavidGrotto.com

Best foods: Fish and vitamin C–rich foods.

The omega-3 fatty acids in fish increase the body's production of inhibitory prostaglandins, substances with anti-inflammatory effects. A recent study found that some patients who consumed fish oil supplements improved so much that they were able to discontinue their use of aspirin, ibuprofen and similar medications.

Ideally, it's best to eat two to three servings of fish a week. Or take a daily fish oil supplement. The usual dose is 1,000 milligrams (mg) to 3,000 mg. Be sure to work with a qualified health professional to determine what supplement regimen is right for you.

Foods rich in vitamin C (citrus fruits, berries, red bell peppers) are effective analgesics because they help decrease joint inflammation. These foods also help protect and repair joint cartilage. A study in *American Journal of Nutrition* found that patients who ate the most vitamin C–rich fruits had 25% lower risk for inflammation.

GOUT

Gout is a form of arthritis that causes severe joint pain that can last for days—and that "flares" at unpredictable intervals.

Weight loss—and avoiding refined carbohydrates, such as white bread, commercially prepared baked goods and other processed foods—can help minimize flare-ups. You also should eat foods that reduce uric acid, a metabolic by-product that causes gout.

Best foods: Celery and cherries.

Celery contains the chemical compound 3-n-butylphthalide, which reduces the body's production of uric acid. Celery also reduces inflammation.

Both sweet (Bing) and tart (Montmorency) pie cherries contain flavonoids, although the bulk of science supporting the anti-inflammatory and pain-relieving properties of cherries has been done using tart cherries. (An exception is the study that found that Bing cherries relieve osteoarthritis.) It is hard to find fresh tart cherries, so I recommend dried tart cherries or tart cherry juice.

MIGRAINES

These debilitating headaches are believed to be caused by the contraction and dilation of blood vessels in the brain.

Best foods: Oats, coffee and tea.

Oats are high in magnesium, a mineral that helps reduce painful muscle spasms—including those in the muscles that line the arteries. In one study, researchers found that people who took 600 mg of magnesium daily had a 41.6% reduction in the number of migraines over a 12-week period, compared with only a 15.8% reduction in those who took a placebo.

You can get plenty of magnesium by eating high-magnesium foods. A small bowl of cooked oat bran (about one cup), for example, provides more than 20% of the daily value. Other high-magnesium foods include oatmeal, almonds, broccoli and pumpkin seeds.

The caffeine in coffee and tea helps relieve migraine pain. The antioxidants in both beverages also are helpful.

Caution: Consuming too much caffeine—or abruptly giving it up if you are a regular coffee or tea drinker—can increase the frequency and severity of headaches. Limit yourself to a few cups daily.

MUSCLE PAIN

It usually is caused by tension, overuse or an actual injury, such as a strain or sprain. Because tendons and ligaments (the tissues that attach your muscles to your bones) have little circulation, muscle-related pain can be very slow to heal.

Best foods: Tart cherries and rose hip tea.

Eating as few as 20 dried tart cherries can help reduce pain. So can tart cherry juice.

Example: At the Sports and Exercise Science Research Centre at London South Bank University, researchers gave one-ounce servings of tart cherry juice twice daily to athletes who did intense workouts. These athletes regained more of their muscle function more quickly than those who didn't drink the juice. Studies also have shown that the juice can reduce muscle pain after exercise.

Rose hip tea is high in vitamin C, as well as anthcyanins and a substance called *galactolipid*—all of which have been shown to combat inflammation and may help ease muscle and joint pain. Have several cups daily.

NERVE PAIN

Inflammation or injury to a nerve can cause a burning, stabbing pain that is difficult to control with medications. Examples of conditions that cause nerve pain include sciatica (pain along the sciatic nerve from the lower spine down the back of the leg) and neuropathy (nerve damage), a painful complication of diabetes.

Best foods: Turmeric, figs and beans.

Turmeric, a yellow-orange spice that commonly is used in Indian and Asian cooking, is a very effective analgesic. Like ginger, it is an anti-inflammatory that has been shown to reduce pain about as well as ibuprofen—and with none of the side effects.

Both figs and beans—along with whole grains and green leafy vegetables—are rich in B-complex vitamins, which are essential for nerve health. One study, which looked at a form of vitamin B-1, found that patients who took as little as 25 mg four times daily had an improvement in neuropathy. Other B vitamins may have similar effects.

Back Pain? You Might Need More of This Vitamin

Vijay Vad, MD, a sports medicine specialist at the Hospital for Special Surgery and assistant professor of rehabilitation medicine at Weill Cornell Medical College, both in New York City. He is also the founder of the Vad Foundation, an organization that supports medical research related to back pain and arthritis, and the author of *Stop Pain: Inflammation Relief for an Active Life.*

What does your backache have to do with the amount of vitamin D in your body? More than you might think, according to recent research.

Here's why: Vitamin D is needed for normal bone metabolism. People who don't produce enough are especially susceptible to low-back pain, possibly because the vertebrae become weakened. Low vitamin D levels also have been linked to hip pain and knee pain.

My advice: Get your vitamin D level tested once a year, particularly if you live in the Northeastern US or the Pacific Northwest. Limited sun exposure in these areas can make it difficult for the body to synthesize enough vitamin D, and it is difficult to get adequate amounts of this vitamin from food.

If your vitamin D level is low (most experts put the optimal blood level between 20 ng/mL and 36 ng/mL), take a daily supplement that provides 1,000 international units (IU) to 2,000 IU…and continue to get tested annually.

5 Best Brain-Boosting Drinks

David Grotto, RD, a registered dietitian and founder and president of Nutrition Housecall, LLC, an Elmhurst, Illinois–based nutrition consulting firm. He is an adviser to Fitness magazine and blogs for the Real Life Nutrition community featured on WebMD. He is author of *The Best Things You Can Eat.*

Some of the easiest-to-prepare brain foods—meaning foods that can preserve and even improve your memory and other cognitive functions—are actually delicious drinks.

You probably already know about green tea, which is high in epigallocatechin-3-gallate (EGCG), a potent compound that appears to protect neurons from age-related damage. *But the following five drinks are scientifically proven to help your brain, too…*

BEET JUICE

Beets are a nutritional powerhouse—and so is the juice. It increases levels of nitric oxide, a blood gas that improves blood flow. How does that help your brain? Your brain needs good blood flow to function optimally.

A recent study looked at brain scans of participants before and after they drank beet juice. The post-beverage scans showed an increase in circulation to the brain's white matter in the frontal lobes—a part of the brain that's often damaged in people with dementia.

You can buy ready-made beet juice at health-food stores, although it's much less expensive to make your own with fresh beets (include the root and greens, which are nutritious as well).

Beet juice has a naturally sweet taste, but you may want to add a little apple juice or another fruit juice—both for flavor and to make the mixture more pourable.

BERRY SMOOTHIES

Acai, a South American fruit that reduces inflammation, is ranked near the top of brain-healthy foods because it dilates blood vessels and increases blood flow.

Its juice has a pleasant taste—something like a cross between raspberry and cocoa—but it's very expensive (typically $30 or more for a quart).

What I recommend: Blend a variety of everyday frozen berries that have been shown to boost brain health—raspberries, blueberries and strawberries, for example—along with a little acai juice (and a bit of any other fruit juice, if you wish) to make an easy, delicious smoothie.

Why use frozen berries? They retain the nutritional benefit of fresh berries—and they're easy to buy and last a long time in the freezer...they give your smoothie a nice texture, which you can vary by adding more or less juice...and they're less expensive than fresh berries if you buy large bags.

CARROT JUICE

The old adage is that carrots are good for the eyes (indeed they are)—but we now know that carrot juice is absolutely great for the brain. Like other deeply colored vegetables (sweet potatoes, kale, red peppers, etc.), carrots are high in beta-carotene, an antioxidant that reduces inflammation—believed to be a factor in brain deterioration.

If you have tried carrot juice but didn't like the taste (it's surprisingly sweet), that's no problem. It is a very good "base" for multi-vegetable juices. (Some choices that are good for covering up the carrot flavor include kale, spinach and other dark greens.)

COCOA

A Harvard/Brigham and Women's Hospital study found that adults who drank two daily cups of cocoa did better on memory tests than those who didn't drink it.

The flavanols (a class of antioxidants) in cocoa relax the endothelial linings of blood vessels and help reduce blood pressure. High blood pressure is a leading risk factor for dementia. The antioxidants in cocoa also reduce the cell-damaging effects of free radicals—this may improve long-term brain health.

Important: Do not go overboard with sugar, though—sugar is not good for your brain (and the jury is still out on artificial sweeteners).

Here's my advice: Buy a brand of unsweetened cocoa powder that is processed to remain high in flavanols. You don't have to buy an expensive specialty brand to get the brain-protecting effects. Most major brands of cocoa powder have respectable levels of cocoa flavanols. I advise against using milk chocolate or chocolate syrup—they typically have the least amount of flavanols and the most sugar.

At first, make your hot cocoa with your usual amount of sugar...then slowly cut back. You'll grow to appreciate the deep and pleasantly bitter true taste of the cocoa itself as less and less sugar stops masking it. As for using milk or water for your cocoa, that's your choice.

RED WINE

Everyone knows that red wine promotes cardiovascular health (easy does it). What you might not know is that red wine has been linked to a lower risk for dementia.

One reason is that people who drink moderate amounts of red wine—up to two glasses a day for men or one glass for women—have an increase in HDL "good" cholesterol. Research from Columbia University has found that people with the highest levels of HDL were less likely to develop dementia than those with the lowest levels.

Want to supercharge the brain-boosting power of your red wine? Make delicious Sangria! You'll get the wine's benefits and extra antioxidants and other nutrients from the fruit.

Sangria is typically made by steeping pieces of fresh fruit—lemon, orange, apple and just about any other fruit you like—in a rich red wine such as Merlot or Cabernet Sauvignon (or a Spanish red if you want to be autentico) and adding sugar and another liquor, such as brandy or rum.

My advice: Skip the sugar and extra liquor, but go ahead and add some orange juice to dilute the wine a bit and add some sweetness.

More from David Grotto, RD...

Best Juice Machines

Here, a juicer and two blenders that I recommend for quality and affordability...

• **Green Star GS-1000 Juice Extractor** uses a low-speed, low-heat system to preserve nutrients from produce. $485, *GreenStar.com*.

• **Ninja Professional Blender** has a powerful 1,100-watt motor and six blades to pulverize produce for drinks with lots of pulp. $100, *NinjaKitchen.com*.

• **Vitamix 5200 is a multipurpose blender** that also chops and churns veggies and fruits into smoothies. Easy 30-second self-cleaning. $449, *Vitamix.com*.

Oranges Provide More Than Just Vitamin C

Do oranges have health benefits that are different from those of clementines and tangerines?

The orange-colored citrus fruits you choose to eat is a matter of personal taste, not nutritional value. Oranges and their smaller cousins—including clementines, mandarin oranges and tangerines—have very similar health benefits. Like other kinds of citrus, they all are rich in antioxidants, including vitamin C and bioflavonoids such as hesperidin and quercetin. These powerful antioxidants help fight cancer...boost immunity...build bone...heal wounds...and improve the body's ability to absorb calcium.

David Grotto, RD, founder and president, Nutritional Housecall, LLC, a nutrition counseling firm based in Elmhurst, Illinois. His newest book is *The Best Things You Can Eat: For Everything from Aches to Zzzz*, the *Definitive Guide to the Nutrition-Packed Foods that Energize, Heal, and Help You Look Great*. DavidGrotto.com

Nutty Protection for Your Heart

Pecans, almonds and walnuts protect the heart. Pecans and walnuts are high in a form of vitamin E called gamma tocopherol... almonds are high in alpha tocopherol. These powerful antioxidants help reduce risk of hardening of the arteries and heart disease. They also lower total and LDL (bad) cholesterol and raise HDL (good) cholesterol.

Best: Eat a moderate-sized handful of nuts every day.

Ella Haddad, DrPH, is associate professor, department of nutrition, School of Public Health, Loma Linda University, Loma Linda, California, and leader of a study published in *Nutrition Research*.

Superfood Spirulina Slows Aging and Prevents Chronic Disease

Jennifer Adler, MS, CN, a certified nutritionist, natural foods chef and adjunct faculty member at Bastyr University, Seattle. She is the founder and owner of Passionate Nutrition, a nutrition practice with offices in eight locations in the Puget Sound area, and co-founder of the International Eating Disorders Institute. PassionateNutrition.com

When you think of a superfood, you probably think of salmon or blueberries—not the algae that floats on the surfaces of lakes, ponds and reservoirs.

But there's a type of blue-green algae that has been used for food and medicine in developing countries for centuries...that NASA has recommended as an ideal food for long-term space missions...that is loaded with health-giving nutrients...and that might be a key component in a diet aimed at staying healthy, reversing chronic disease and slowing the aging process.

That algae is spirulina.

Spirulina grows mainly in subtropical and tropical countries, where there is year-round heat and sunlight. It is high in protein (up to 70%), rich in antioxidants and loaded with vitamins and minerals, particularly iron and vitamin B-12. And it has no cellulose—the cell wall of green plants—so its nutrients are easy for the body to digest and absorb.

GREEN MEDICINE

Dried into a powder, spirulina can be added to food or taken as a tablet or capsule. And ingested regularly, spirulina can do you a lot of good. *Scientific research shows there are many health problems that spirulina might help prevent or treat...*

•**Anemia.** Researchers from the University of California at Davis studied 40 people age 50 and older who had been diagnosed with anemia (iron deficiency), giving them a spirulina supplement every day for three months. The study participants had a steady rise in levels of hemoglobin, the iron-carrying component of red blood cells, along with several other factors that indicated increased levels of iron.

•**Weakened immunity.** In the UC Davis study mentioned above, most of the participants ages 61 to 70 also had increases in infection-fighting white blood cells and in an enzyme that is a marker for increased immune activity—in effect, reversing immunosenescence, the age-related weakening of the immune system. Immunosenescence is linked not only to a higher risk for infectious diseases such as the flu but also to chronic diseases with an inflammatory component, such as heart disease, Alzheimer's and cancer.

•**Allergies.** Spirulina has anti-inflammatory properties and can prevent the release of histamine and other inflammatory factors that trigger and worsen allergic symptoms. Studies also show that spirulina can boost levels of IgA, an antibody that defends against allergic reactions. In one study, people with allergies who took spirulina had less nasal discharge, sneezing, nasal congestion and itching.

•**Cataracts and age-related macular degeneration.** Taking spirulina can double blood levels of zeaxanthin, an antioxidant linked to a reduced risk for cataracts and age-related macular degeneration, reported researchers in *British Medical Journal*.

•**Diabetes.** In several studies, researchers found that adding spirulina to the diets of people with type 2 diabetes significantly decreased blood sugar levels.

Caution: Spirulina has not been approved by the FDA for treating diabetes, so consult your doctor before taking.

•**Lack of endurance.** In a small study, men who took spirulina for one month were able to run more than 30% longer on a treadmill before having to stop because of fatigue, reported Greek researchers in Medicine & Science in Sports & Exercise.

•**Heart disease.** Nearly a dozen studies have looked at the effect of spirulina intake on risk factors for heart disease, both in healthy people and people with heart disease. Most of the studies found significant decreases in negative factors (such as LDL cholesterol, total cholesterol, triglycerides, apolipoprotein B and blood pressure) and increases in positive factors (such as HDL cholesterol and apolipoprotein A1).

IDEAL DOSE

A preventive daily dose of spirulina is one teaspoon. A therapeutic dose, to control or reverse disease, is 10 grams, or one tablespoon.

Spirulina has been on the market for more than a decade, and it's among the substances listed by the FDA as "Generally Recognized as Safe" (GRAS).

Caution: If you have an autoimmune disease, such as multiple sclerosis, rheumatoid arthritis or lupus, talk to your doctor. Spirulina could stimulate the immune system, making the condition worse.

BEST PRODUCTS

Like many products, the quality of spirulina varies. What to look for...

•**Clean taste.** Top-quality spirulina tastes fresh. If spirulina tastes fishy or "swampy" or has a lingering aftertaste, it's probably not a good product.

•**Bright color.** Spirulina should have a vibrant, bright blue-green appearance (more green than blue). If spirulina is olive-green, it's probably inferior.

•**Cost.** You get what you pay for—and good spirulina can be somewhat pricey.

Example: Spirulina Pacifica, from Nutrex Hawaii—grown on the Kona coast of Hawaii since 1984 and regarded by many health experts as one of the most nutritious and purest spirulina products on the market—costs $50 for a 16-ounce, 454-gram jar of powder. Store it in the refrigerator.

•**Growing location.** The best spirulina is grown in clean water in a nonindustrialized setting, as far away as possible from an urban, polluted environment. If you can, find out the growing location of the product you're considering buying.

HOW TO ADD IT TO FOOD

There are many ways to include spirulina in your daily diet…

•**Put it in smoothies.** Add between one teaspoon and one tablespoon to any smoothie or shake.

•**Add to juice.** Add one teaspoon or tablespoon to an eight-ounce glass of juice or water, shake it up and drink it.

•**Sprinkle it on food.** Try spirulina popcorn, for instance—a great conversation starter at a potluck. To a bowl of popcorn, add one to two tablespoons of spirulina powder, three to four tablespoons of grated Parmesan cheese, two or three tablespoons of olive oil, one-half teaspoon of salt and one-eighth teaspoon of cayenne pepper.

•**Add it to condiments.** Put one-quarter teaspoon in a small jar of ketchup, barbecue sauce, mustard or salad dressing. This way you'll get a little each time you use these products.

Watermelon Prevents Sore Muscles

Encarna Aguayo, PhD, associate professor, department of food engineering, Universidad Politécnica de Cartagena, Spain. Her study was published in *Journal of Agricultural and Food Chemistry*.

Don't you love how great it feels to take a hike, hit the gym, do some yard work or otherwise move your muscles? And don't you hate how sore your poor muscles feel the next day? Ah, if only there were a way to get a good workout without suffering the after-aches.

There is, a recent study suggests…and it's not only simple and economical, it's tasty, too.

The secret weapon: Watermelon.

Though watermelon has a reputation for being mostly, well, water—plus natural sugar—it's actually pretty nutritious. Watermelon is high in vitamins A and C…ounce for ounce, it contains more of the powerful antioxidant lycopene than the much touted tomato…and it is one of only a few foods that provides L-citrulline, an amino acid our kidneys use to make arginine, a powerful vasodilator that can improve blood flow.

Some studies suggest that L-citrulline boosts athletic performance by increasing the amount of oxygen brought to muscles during exercise, which is why L-citrulline supplements are marketed for athletes. The study, however, suggests that there's a better way than supplements to get your L-citrulline…and that soreness prevention rather than performance enhancement is the true benefit.

FROM LAB TO GYM

The first part of the study took place in the laboratory, with the purpose of determining L-citrulline's bioavailability. Cells that mimicked the construction and function of the lining of human intestines were placed in petri dishes and exposed to one of three concoctions…

•**Natural watermelon juice,** made by liquefying watermelon pulp in a juicer (this is basically what winds up in your digestive tract after you eat watermelon).

• **Watermelon juice that had been pasteurized by heating it to 175°F for 40 seconds** (as commercially available bottled watermelon juice typically is to increase its shelf life).

• **An L-citrulline supplement mixed with water.**

The researchers then measured the amount of L-citrulline that was absorbed by the intestine-like cells.

Findings: Natural watermelon juice had a significantly higher absorption rate (18.87%) than the pasteurized juice (13.19%) or the supplement (11.85%)—meaning that the unadulterated watermelon juice provided the most bioavailable form of L-citrulline.

The next part of the study took place in a gym. Participants included physically active young men who, over the course of two weeks, performed the same exercise routine three times. Each time, one hour before starting their workouts, they drank 17 ounces of either natural, unpasteurized watermelon juice (containing 1.17 grams of L-citrulline)... unpasteurized watermelon juice enriched with extra L-citrulline (for a total of 6.0 grams of L-citrulline)...or a placebo drink (an infusion of fruits and other plants that did not contain L-citrulline). All of the drinks looked alike and had the same natural sugar content. Participants were not told what the drinks contained or what effects the researchers were looking for.

The men wore heart rate monitors while riding stationary bikes at a very heavy resistance setting. They periodically rated their perceived exertion levels during the workouts...and reported their degree of muscle soreness 24 hours and 48 hours after completing the exercise routines. Each participant did the workout on three separate occasions so that everyone's reaction to each drink could be measured.

Results: Participants reported significantly less muscle soreness 24 hours after drinking watermelon juice than after drinking the placebo concoction. (After 48 hours, soreness levels were minimal no matter which drink was consumed.) Interestingly, post-exercise soreness ratings were the same with the natural watermelon juice as with the enriched watermelon juice—suggesting that the unadulterated juice provided enough L-citrulline to reduce muscle soreness, and that the extra dose of L-citrulline in the enriched juice did not provide any additional benefit.

Surprisingly, given L-citrulline's reputation as a performance enhancer, there were no differences in cycling speed, heart rate or perceived exertion no matter which drink the participants consumed before their workouts. However, it's possible that consuming watermelon might enhance performance not on the same day, but rather on subsequent days, by making your muscles less sore and therefore allowing you to work out harder. It's also possible that, if you consistently consume watermelon, then this performance boost might be ongoing. Further research would be needed to explore that theory...and also to determine how helpful watermelon juice might be for other types of people, such as women, for novice exercises or for elite athletes. These researchers hope to do additional studies on watermelon juice in the near future.

In the meantime, though, if you're anticipating a strenuous workout, why not pull out your juicer and make some watermelon juice or just eat some watermelon before you exert yourself to see if this keeps your muscles from aching afterward? To get the same 1.17 grams of L-citrulline used in the study, you would need to drink 17 ounces of watermelon juice...or eat about four cups of cut-up watermelon cubes.

Chicken Soup With a Healing Kick!

J.E. Williams, OMD, is a naturopathic doctor, acupuncturist and doctor of Oriental medicine. He is the author of *Beating the Flu and Viral Immunity*. DrJEWilliams.com

Whether you've got a bad cold or the flu, chicken soup is the ultimate comfort food. And its healing effects are more than folklore. Research shows that chicken soup does seem to have anti-inflammatory properties that help fight infection.

For even more healing power: Add flavorful, spicy foods that attack germs and help control nasal congestion…and spices with antiviral effects.

Helpful: The soup can be frozen for up to three months.

Ingredients:

1 5-lb whole chicken

6 chopped garlic cloves

1 medium-sized, peeled gingerroot

12 large carrots

6 celery stalks

3 medium white or yellow potatoes

3 large red onions

2 green or red jalapeño peppers

1 bunch parsley

1 bunch fresh oregano

(or 1 teaspoon dried oregano)

1 bunch fresh rosemary

(or 1 teaspoon dried rosemary)

1 bunch fresh sage

(or 1 teaspoon dried sage)

Put the chicken in a large pot, and cover with cold water. Bring to a boil. Add garlic and ginger. Simmer for 60 minutes. (Skim some of the fat off as it cooks.) Add chopped carrots, celery, potatoes and onions. Simmer for 45 additional minutes. Remove chicken, and pull meat from the bones. Return meat to the pot, and add chopped jalapeño peppers (without the seeds) and parsley, oregano, rosemary and sage. Cook another 15 minutes. Add black pepper (it helps clear mucus), and lightly salt to taste. Enjoy!

Healthier Potatoes and Pasta

Study of resistant starch content of potatoes by cooking method presented by researchers at the USDA Agricultural Research Service (ARS) Grand Forks Human Nutrition Research Center, North Dakota, and the University of Minnesota, Minneapolis and St. Paul, at the Federation of American Societies for Experimental Biology conference in Boston.

Study titled "Efficacy of increased resistant starch consumption in human type 2 diabetes" by researchers at University of Surrey, United Kingdom, published in *Endocrine Connections*.

I s there a healthy way to cook potatoes and pasta? The answer is yes…but how much healthier is open to debate.

Let's take a 100-gram serving of potatoes—about three-and-a-half ounces. Boil it, and you've got 2.6 grams of resistant starch…baked, 3.1 grams…chilled (either baked or boiled), 4.3 grams—good news for potato salad lovers. Chilled and then reheated potatoes do pretty well, too—3.5 grams. The same holds true for pasta—cooking and then cooling pasta increases the resistant starch modestly.

Does it make a difference? In a British study, people with diabetes who added 40 grams of resistant starch to their daily intake didn't improve their underlying diabetes but did have a reduced blood sugar spike after meals—a healthy thing. Whether there's any blood sugar benefit to taking in, say, an additional two or three grams of resistant starch in a meal, though, just isn't known.

So go ahead and enjoy your potatoes baked rather than boiled, and even better yet, cooled. But remember these foods already start with lots of easily digested, sugar-spiking starch, so cooking them in a way that boosts their resistant starch doesn't turn them into superfoods. A baked Russet Burbank potato has a "glycemic index" (GI), a measure of how quickly it raises blood sugar, of 111—more than white bread. So cook it right, but don't make it a daily staple—and add a healthful fat, such as olive oil, to further lower the GI.

Pasta, on the other hand, already has a lower GI than spuds, because the way it's made traps starch in a matrix that takes the body a longer time to break down into sugar. The GI range—30 to 60. So enjoy your pasta cooled in pasta salads...and if you like it hot, reduce its GI even more by cooking it al dente—slightly chewy rather than soft—and drizzling it with olive oil.

In the end, though, what matters more is how much you eat of these delicious but high-starch foods. Want to make a really healthy pasta salad? Start with whole grain pasta for extra nutrition, cook it al dente, and use just one cup of cooled pasta with three cups of chopped nonstarchy veggies with your favorite dressing. Now you're cooking.

Eat This Fruit to Lower Cholesterol

Bahram H. Arjmandi, PhD, RD, Margaret A. Sitton Professor, chair, department of nutrition, food, and exercise sciences, director Center for Advancing Exercise and Nutrition Research on Aging, The Florida State University, Tallahassee. The results of his study were published in *Journal of the Academy of Nutrition and Dietetics.*

Sure, statin drugs such as Lipitor and Zocor can be effective in bringing down elevated cholesterol—and, therefore, your risk for heart disease—but these benefits come at a price.

Side effects of these powerful drugs can include raised blood sugar, memory loss and muscle damage.

Seeking a safer, natural solution to at least supplement (if not fully replace) statins, scientists recently looked at the impact of two fruits on cholesterol.

And the results were quite promising—especially for one of the fruits.

TASTES GOOD...LESS CHOLESTEROL

In the study, researchers asked participants—all women—to eat a half cup of dried apples or a half cup of dried plums (prunes) each day for a year. The study did not include people who had regularly consumed dried apples or prunes in the past or anyone who was taking cholesterol-lowering drugs. Participants were asked to eat whatever else they typically ate and to

exercise the same amount that they normally would. Roughly the same percentage of people in each group—about 82%—complied with all the instructions and completed the study. And the results below are based only on those who complied and completed the study.

Cholesterol levels were checked at the beginning of the study and after three months, six months and 12 months. *Results...*

• **After three months.** Those who ate dried apples reduced their total cholesterol by 9% and their LDL "bad" cholesterol by 16%...while those who ate prunes reduced their total cholesterol by only 2.6% and their LDL by just 5%.

• **After six months.** Those who ate dried apples reduced their numbers even more—their total cholesterol dropped by 13% and their LDL by 24%, compared with levels at the beginning of the study. But the prune group's levels didn't change between the three-month mark and the six-month mark.

• **After 12 months.** The dried-apple group's results were the same as they were at the six-month mark. The prune group saw a little more improvement at this point—their total cholesterol was 3.5% lower and LDL was 8% lower, compared with levels at the beginning of the study.

In other words, overall, it seems that both dried apples and prunes brought down cholesterol, but dried apples had a stronger effect. Though this study looked only at women, the researchers believe that the results are likely to apply to men as well.

Though head-to-head fruit versus statin studies haven't been done, neither fruit is likely to lower cholesterol quite as much as a statin would (depending on the dose, a statin tends to lower LDL by roughly 40% to 60%). But given that they're natural foods that provide excellent nutrition and no harmful side effects, this news is quite encouraging.

THE PECTIN PUNCH

Both dried fruits offer heart-healthy antioxidant and anti-inflammatory protection and are rich in pectin—a dietary fiber that reduces cholesterol, said Bahram H. Arjmandi, PhD, RD, lead investigator of the study. Dried apples helped more, probably, because apples (both dried and fresh) contain an especially high amount of pectin.

In case you're wondering, dried apples (rather than regular, fresh apples) were studied for the sake of consistency. Since there are significant variations in the chemical composition of fresh fruits, studying dried apples was a more standardized way to measure their effects. But fresh apples, said Dr. Arjmandi, are apt to provide the same cholesterol-lowering benefits as dried apples. To eat an amount of fresh apples that is equal to what the study subjects ate through dried apples (one-half cup), you would need to eat two medium-sized fresh apples per day.

To try: Slice fresh apples and dip them in peanut butter…blend some into your lunchtime smoothie…or sprinkle cinnamon on them and eat them as a sweet after-dinner treat.

On the other hand, dried apples are easier to transport and store and they keep much longer—so it's easy to keep them around for snacking. You can also use dried apples as a garnish and add them to cereal, yogurt, soup or pasta dishes. (Try it!)

If you do so and you also take a statin, said Dr. Arjmandi, continue seeing your doctor to track your cholesterol, because it may turn out that you can reduce your statin dose—and that would be sweet.

---

5 Foods That Fight High Blood Pressure (You Might Not Even Need Medication)

Janet Bond Brill, PhD, RD, a nationally recognized nutrition, health and fitness expert who specializes in cardiovascular disease prevention. She has authored several books on the topic, including *Blood Pressure DOWN, Prevent a Second Heart Attack* and *Cholesterol DOWN*. DrJanet.com

Is your blood pressure on the high side? Your doctor might write a prescription when it creeps above 140/90—but you may be able to forgo medication. Lifestyle changes still are considered the best starting treatment for mild hypertension. These include not smoking, regular exercise and a healthy diet. *In addition to eating less salt, you want to include potent pressure-lowering foods, including…*

RAISINS

Raisins are basically dehydrated grapes, but they provide a much more concentrated dose of nutrients and fiber. They are high in potassium, with 220 milligrams (mg) in a small box (1.5 ounces). Potassium helps counteract the blood pressure–raising effects of salt. The more potassium we consume, the more sodium our bodies excrete. Researchers also speculate that the fiber and antioxidants in raisins change the biochemistry of blood vessels, making them more pliable—important for healthy blood pressure. Opt for dark raisins over light-colored ones because dark raisins have more catechins, a powerful type of antioxidant that can increase blood flow.

Researchers at Louisville Metabolic and Atherosclerosis Research Center compared people who snacked on raisins with those who ate other packaged snacks. Those in the raisin group had drops in systolic pressure (the top number) ranging from 4.8 points (after four weeks) to 10.2 points (after 12 weeks). Blood pressure barely budged in the no-raisin group. Some people worry about the sugar in raisins, but it is natural sugar (not added sugar) and will not adversely affect your health (though people with diabetes need to be cautious with portion sizes).

My advice: Aim to consume a few ounces of raisins every day. Prunes are an alternative.

BEETS

Beets, too, are high in potassium, with about 519 mg per cup. They're delicious, easy to cook (see the tasty recipe below) and very effective for lowering blood pressure.

A study at The London Medical School found that people who drank about eight ounces of beet juice averaged a 10-point drop in blood pressure during the next 24 hours. The blood pressure–lowering effect was most pronounced at three to six hours past drinking but remained lower for the entire 24 hours. Eating whole beets might be even better because you will get extra fiber.

Along with fiber and potassium, beets also are high in nitrate. The nitrate is converted first to nitrite in the blood, then to nitric oxide. Nitric oxide is a gas that relaxes blood vessel walls and lowers blood pressure.

My advice: Eat beets several times a week. Look for beets that are dark red. They contain more protective phytochemicals than the gold or white beets. Cooked spinach and kale are alternatives.

DAIRY

In research involving nearly 45,000 people, researchers found that those who consumed low-fat "fluid" dairy foods, such as yogurt and low-fat milk, were 16% less likely to develop high blood pressure. Higher-fat forms of dairy, such as cheese and ice cream, had no blood pressure benefits. The study was published in *Journal of Human Hypertension*.

In another study, published in *The New England Journal of Medicine*, researchers found that people who included low-fat or fat-free dairy in a diet high in fruits and vegetables had double the blood pressure–lowering benefits of those who just ate the fruits and veggies.

Low-fat dairy is high in calcium, another blood pressure–lowering mineral that should be included in your diet. When you don't have enough calcium in your diet, a "calcium leak" occurs in your kidneys. This means that the kidneys excrete more calcium in the urine, disturbing the balance of mineral metabolism involved in blood pressure regulation.

My advice: Aim for at least one serving of low-fat or nonfat milk or yogurt every day. If you don't care for cow's milk or can't drink it, switch to fortified soy milk. It has just as much calcium and protein and also contains phytoestrogens, compounds that are good for the heart.

FLAXSEED

Flaxseed contains alpha-linolenic acid (ALA), an omega-3 fatty acid that helps prevent heart and vascular disease. Flaxseed also contains magnesium. A shortage of magnesium in our diet throws off the balance of sodium, potassium and calcium, which causes the blood vessels to constrict.

Flaxseed also is high in flavonoids, the same antioxidants that have boosted the popularity of dark chocolate, kale and red wine. Flavonoids are bioactive chemicals that reduce inflammation throughout the body, including in the arteries. Arterial inflammation is thought to be the "trigger" that leads to high blood pressure, blood clots and heart attacks.

In a large-scale observational study linking dietary magnesium intake with better heart health and longevity, nearly 59,000 healthy Japanese people were followed for 15 years. The scientists found that the people with the highest dietary intake of magnesium had a 50% reduced risk for death from heart disease (heart attack and stroke). According to the researchers, magnesium's heart-healthy benefit is linked to its ability to improve blood pressure, suppress irregular heartbeats and inhibit inflammation.

My advice: Add one or two tablespoons of ground flaxseed to breakfast cereals. You also can sprinkle flaxseed on yogurt or whip it into a breakfast smoothie. Or try chia seeds.

WALNUTS

Yale researchers found that people who ate two ounces of walnuts a day had improved blood flow and drops in blood pressure (a 3.5-point drop in systolic blood pressure and a 2.8-point drop in diastolic blood pressure). The mechanisms through which walnuts elicit a blood pressure–lowering response are believed to involve their high content of monounsaturated fatty acids, omega-3 ALA, magnesium and fiber, and their low levels of sodium and saturated fatty acids.

Bonus: Despite the reputation of nuts as a "fat snack," the people who ate them didn't gain weight.

The magnesium in walnuts is particularly important. It limits the amount of calcium that enters muscle cells inside artery walls. Ingesting the right amount of calcium (not too much and not too little) on a daily basis is essential for optimal blood pressure regulation. Magnesium regulates calcium's movement across the membranes of the smooth muscle cells, deep within the artery walls.

If your body doesn't have enough magnesium, too much calcium will enter the smooth muscle cells, which causes the arterial muscles to tighten, putting a squeeze on the arteries and raising blood pressure. Magnesium works like the popular calcium channel blockers, drugs that block entry of calcium into arterial walls, lowering blood pressure.

My advice: Eat two ounces of walnuts every day. Or choose other nuts such as almonds and pecans.

DR. JANET'S ROASTED RED BEETS
WITH LEMON VINAIGRETTE

Beets are a delicious side dish when roasted, peeled and topped with a lemony vinaigrette and fresh parsley. This recipe is from my book *Prevent a Second Heart Attack.*

- 6 medium-sized beets, washed and trimmed of greens and roots
- 2 Tablespoons extra-virgin olive oil
- 2 teaspoons fresh lemon juice
- 1 garlic clove, peeled and minced
- 1 teaspoon Dijon mustard
- ¼ teaspoon kosher salt
- ¼ teaspoon freshly ground black pepper
- ¼ cup chopped fresh flat-leaf Italian parsley

Preheat the oven to 400°F. Spray a baking dish with nonstick cooking spray. Place the beets in the dish, and cover tightly with foil. Bake the beets for about one hour or until they are tender when pierced with a fork or thin knife. Remove from the oven, and allow to cool to the touch.

Meanwhile, in a small bowl, whisk together the olive oil, lemon juice, garlic, mustard, salt and pepper for the dressing. When the beets are cool enough to handle, peel and slice the beets, arranging the slices on a platter. Drizzle with vinaigrette, and garnish with parsley. Serves six.

Six Ways to Liven Up Your Heart-Healthy Diet

Janet Bond Brill, PhD, RD, an expert in nutrition and cardiovascular disease prevention based in Valley Forge, Pennsylvania. She is director of nutrition for Fitness Together, a franchise company of almost 500 personal fitness-training studios, has served as a nutrition consultant for several corporations and is the author of *Prevent a Second Heart Attack.* DrJanet.com

Just about everyone knows that a Mediterranean-style diet can help prevent heart disease. Even if you've already had a heart attack, this style of eating—emphasizing such foods as fish and vegetables—can reduce the risk for a second heart attack by up to 70%.

Problem: About 80% of patients with heart disease quit following dietary advice within one year after their initial diagnosis. That's often because they want more choices but aren't sure which foods have been proven to work.

Solution: Whether you already have heart disease or want to prevent it, you can liven up your diet by trying foods that usually don't get much attention for their heart-protective benefits…

SECRET 1: **Popcorn.** It's more than just a snack. It's a whole grain that's high in cholesterol-lowering fiber. Surprisingly, popcorn contains more fiber, per ounce, than whole-wheat bread or brown rice.

Scientific evidence: Data from the 1999–2002 National Health and Nutrition Examination Survey found that people who eat popcorn daily get 22% more fiber than those who don't eat it.

Important: Eat "natural" popcorn, preferably air-popped or microwaved in a brown paper bag, without added oil. The commercially prepared popcorn packets generally contain too much salt, butter and other additives. Three cups of popped popcorn, which contain almost 6 g of fiber and 90 calories, is considered a serving of whole grains. Studies have shown that at least three servings of whole grains a day (other choices include oatmeal and brown rice) may help reduce the risk for heart disease, high cholesterol and obesity.

SECRET 2: **Chia seeds.** You're probably familiar with Chia pets—those terra-cotta figures that sprout thick layers of grassy "fur." The same seeds, native to Mexico and Guatemala, are increasingly available in health-food stores. I consider them a superfood because they have a nutrient profile that rivals heart-healthy flax-seed.

In fact, chia seeds contain more omega-3 fatty acids than flaxseed. Omega-3s increase the body's production of anti-inflammatory eicosanoids, hormonelike substances that help prevent "adhesion molecules" from causing plaque buildup and increasing atherosclerosis.

Scientific evidence: A study published in the *Journal of the American College of Cardiology*, which looked at nearly 40,000 participants, found that an omega-3 rich diet can prevent and even reverse existing cardiovascular disease.

Other benefits: One ounce of chia seeds has 10 g of fiber, 5 g of alpha-linolenic acid and 18% of the Recommended Dietary Allowance for calcium for adults ages 19 to 50.

Chia seeds look and taste something like poppy seeds. You can add them to baked goods, such as muffins, or sprinkle them on salads and oatmeal or other cereals.

SECRET 3: **Figs.** They're extraordinarily rich in antioxidants with an oxygen radical absorbance capacity (ORAC) score of 3,383. Scientists use this ORAC scale to determine the antioxidant capacity of various foods. An orange, by comparison, scores only about 1,819. Fresh figs are among the best sources of beta-carotene and other heart-healthy carotenoids.

Scientific evidence: In a study published in the *Journal of the American College of Nutrition*, two groups of participants were "challenged" with sugary soft drinks, which are known to increase arterial oxidation. Oxidation in the arteries triggers atherosclerosis, a main risk factor for heart disease. Those who were given only soda had a drop in healthful antioxidant activity in the blood...those who were given figs as well as soda had an increase in blood antioxidant levels.

Bonus: Ten dried figs contain 140 mg of calcium. Other compounds in figs, such as quercetin, reduce inflammation and dilate the arteries. Perhaps for these reasons, people who eat figs regularly have much less heart disease than those who don't eat them, according to studies.

Most dried figs contain added sulfites, so it's best to buy organic, sulfite-free dried figs.

SECRET 4: **Soy protein.** Tofu, soy milk and other soy foods are "complete proteins"—that is, they supply all of the essential amino acids that your body needs but without the cholesterol and large amount of saturated fat found in meat.

Scientific evidence: People who replace dairy or meat protein with soy will have an average drop in LDL "bad" cholesterol of 2% to 7%, according to research from the American Heart Association. Every 1% drop in LDL lowers heart disease risk about 2%.

A one-half cup serving of tofu provides 10 g of protein. An eight-ounce glass of soy milk gives about 7 g. Edamame (steamed or boiled green soybeans) has about 9 g per half cup. Avoid processed soy products, such as hydrogenated soybean oil (a trans fat), soy isoflavone powders and soy products with excess added sodium.

SECRET 5: **Lentils.** I call these "longevity legumes" because studies have shown that they can literally extend your life.

Best choices: **Brown or black lentils.**

Scientific evidence: In one study, published in the *Asia Pacific Journal of Clinical Nutrition*, the eating habits of five groups of older adults were compared. For every 20 g (a little less than three-fourths of an ounce) increase in the daily intake of lentils and/or other legumes, there was an 8% reduction in the risk of dying within seven years.

Lentils contain large amounts of fiber, plant protein and antioxidants along with folate, iron and magnesium—all of which are important for cardiovascular health.

Similarly, a Harvard study found that people who ate one serving of cooked beans (one-third cup) a day were 38% less likely to have a heart attack than those who ate beans less than once a month.

Caution: Beans have been shown to cause gout flare-ups in some people.

Important: Lentils cook much faster than other beans. They don't need presoaking. When simmered in water, they're ready in 20 to 30 minutes. You need about one-half cup of cooked lentils, beans or peas each day for heart health.

SECRET 6: **Pinot Noir and Cabernet Sauvignon.** All types of alcohol seem to have some heart-protective properties, but red wine offers the most.

Scientific evidence: People who drink alcohol regularly in moderation (one five-ounce glass of wine daily for women, and no more than two for men) have a 30% to 50% lower risk of dying from a heart attack than those who don't drink, according to research published in *Archives of Internal Medicine*.

Best choices: Pinot Noir, Cabernet Sauvignon and Tannat wines (made from Tannat red grapes). These wines have the highest concentrations of flavonoids, antioxidants that reduce arterial inflammation and inhibit the oxidation of LDL cholesterol. Oxidation is the process that makes cholesterol more likely to accumulate within artery walls.

Bonus: Red wines also contain resveratrol, a type of polyphenol that is thought to increase the synthesis of proteins that slow aging. Red wine has 10 times more polyphenols than white varieties.

In a four-year study of nearly 7,700 men and women nondrinkers, those who began to drink a moderate amount of red wine cut their risk for heart attack by 38% compared with nondrinkers.

If you are a nondrinker or currently drink less than the amounts described above, talk to your doctor before changing your alcohol intake. If you cannot drink alcohol, pomegranate or purple grape juice is a good alternative.

Saffron Fights Pancreatic Cancer...and Much More

Study titled "Crocetinic acid inhibits hedgehog signaling to inhibit pancreatic cancer stem cells" by researchers at University of Kansas Medical Center, Kansas City, and University of Pune, India, published in *Oncotarget*.

The aromatic spice saffron is worth more by weight than gold. For people with pancreatic cancer, it may someday be even more valuable. At the University of Kansas Medical Center, investigators have found that crocetinic acid, derived from crocetin, an active ingredient in saffron that helps gives the spice its bright red-orange color, strongly inhibits pancreatic cancer in mice. In the study, crocetinic acid targeted and inhibited pancreatic stem cells—which often elude conventional chemotherapy and cause pancreatic cancer to spread. Even at high doses, crocetinic acid showed no toxic effect on normal cells. While much more research, including human studies, is needed before the compound can become a cancer drug, the work is exciting because a nontoxic chemotherapeutic agent against pancreatic cancer is desperately needed—it is the fourth-leading cause of cancer deaths in the US and one of the most lethal of all cancers.

The new research was done with a purified substance that is 50 times more concentrated than crocetin, so we don't know if cooking with saffron or taking saffron supplements can fight cancer. But we already know that the spice is extraordinarily healthful. It has powerful antioxidant and anti-inflammatory effects, protects nerve cells, improves cardiovascular function, enhances memory, reduces anxiety and protects eyesight. Clinical studies have found that saffron supplements slow the progression of the eye disease macular degeneration...and in some cases treat clinical depression just as well as common antidepressants such as *fluoxetine* (Prozac).

The typical dose in those studies is 30 mg a day, usually taken in two divided doses. That is about as much you would get in a saffron-infused dish—the classic Spanish dish paella, for example, which uses one-quarter of a gram (that is, 250 mg) to feed eight people. Yes, it's an expensive spice, but it takes only a tiny amount to spread its aromatic beauty to a dish—and enhance health. You can even use it to make a mood-boosting tea.

A note about safety and quality: Although saffron supplements appear to be very safe, very large doses can be toxic—do not exceed 1,500 mg, which is far above the therapeutic dose used in studies. Also, powdered culinary saffron may be adulterated with cheaper spices such as turmeric or marigold petals—a better bet is to buy saffron threads. (*Note*: Saffron threads are available at *BottomLine Store.com*.)

Are Your Grandmother's Prunes the New Superfood?

Maria Stacewicz-Sapuntzakis, PhD, professor emerita, department of kinesiology and nutrition, University of Illinois at Chicago.

What comes to mind when you hear the word "prunes"? You probably think of two things—laxatives or senior citizens. That's why the prune industry is trying to change the name to "dried plums." But the fact is, prunes are amazingly good for us. They are nutrient-rich...inexpensive...they can satisfy a sweet tooth without the horrid effects of processed sugar...they can even help you get going with a healthy slimming diet. *But there's a lot more to this simple, inexpensive superfood—yes, superfood—that could make you healthier and get you thinking about prunes in a whole new way...*

A MAGIC INGREDIENT

Prunes have a unique combination of nutrients that aren't found in other foods, not even other dried fruits. They're very high in a sugar alcohol called sorbitol, which is the key magic ingredient to the prune's health benefits.

On its own, too much dietary sorbitol can cause gas and unwanted laxative effects, and 50 grams or more a day is considered excessive. In fact, the FDA makes companies add warning labels about the laxative effect of sorbitol to food products that contain it. But you'd have to eat more than half a pound of prunes in one sitting to total 50 grams—and if you try that at home, you sure will be "sitting." Five prunes contain a modest 7 grams of sorbitol and the sorbitol in prunes combines with other nutrients in the fruit to pump up its nutritional and health-enhancing powers.

According to Dr. Stacewicz-Sapuntzakis, two daily servings of prunes (that's 10 to 12) can help your body...

• **Lose weight.** Despite the fact that they average 25 calories each, snacking on prunes can help you lose weight. Research reported at the European Congress on Obesity found that dieters who ate prunes lost more pounds and more inches and felt fuller longer than dieters who didn't eat them. The finding on satiety matched earlier research that found that eating prunes as a mid-morning snack can help you eat less at lunchtime.

• **Regulate blood sugar.** Although prunes are sweet, they rate relatively low on the Glycemic Index scale, which measures how fast and how much a certain food raises blood sugar levels. This makes prunes a good food choice for folks with hyperglycemia or diabetes. Sorbitol itself has a low glycemic value, which may explain why something that tastes so much like candy keeps blood sugar levels on an even keel instead of making them spike.

• **Strengthen bones.** Prunes contain several nutrients, including boron, copper, vitamin K and, as mentioned, potassium that help prevent bone loss. Plus, sorbitol—that secret ingredient—increases absorption of calcium from prunes and other foods.

• **Prevent or slow arteriosclerosis.** Studies in animals and humans suggest that compounds in prunes can lower blood levels of cholesterol and, thereby, prevent or slow the progression of arteriosclerosis—or hardening of the arteries—caused by buildup of cholesterol and other debris on artery walls.

• **Prevent colon cancer.** The fiber, phenolic compounds (which are antioxidant substances found in fruits) and sorbitol help prunes move waste through the colon quickly enough to keep bile acid by-products from injuring the lining of the colon, which can be cancer-causing.

THE BEST WAYS TO EAT PRUNES

Is drinking prune juice just as good as eating prunes? If you eat the whole fruit, you get the benefits of all the great nutritional compounds in prunes. Some of these compounds become lost in prune juice. But if you have never eaten prunes and now have an interest in adding them to your diet, start slow with four or five a day. Once you're sure that your body can tolerate them without an unwanted laxative effect, work up to 10 to 12 each day. That racks up 240 calories, but you'll feel full longer than if you ate the same amount of calories in the form of, say, bread and cheese.

And prunes can be a lot more than wrinkled things you pluck from a box. *Consider these tasty ways to enjoy them…*

•**Homemade no-bake energy bars.** Place a handful of prunes in a food processor along with any combination of your favorite nuts and seeds, such as almonds, walnuts, and sesame, sunflower or pumpkin seeds. You can add some shredded coconut, too…maybe even sprinkle in some unsweetened cacao to sate a chocolate craving. Process the ingredients into a paste, and then press the mixture into a baking dish. Chill until firm and cut into squares for a perfect on-the-go energy boost and healthy sweet-tooth satisfier.

•**Prunes in a Blanket.** Wrap individual prunes in paper-thin slices of prosciutto—or do the same using turkey bacon if you prefer—then roast at 400°F until crisp on the outside, sweet and gooey inside.

•**Spicy Moroccan-Style Stew.** Simmer prunes with lamb, beef or chicken and aromatic Moroccan spices, such as ginger, saffron, cinnamon and pepper, to serve up a traditional Moroccan stew called tagine.

Bon appétit and healthy eating with prunes!

The Diet That Makes Menopause a Breeze

Holly Lucille, ND, RN, a naturopathic doctor based in West Hollywood, California. She is the author of *Creating and Maintaining Balance: A Woman's Guide to Safe, Natural Hormone Health* and serves on the board of directors for the Institute for Natural Medicine. DrHollyLucille.com

How does diet affect the annoying symptoms of menopause? Bottom Line/HEALTH spoke with naturopath Holly Lucille to find out.

Holly Lucille, ND, RN: When it comes to menopause, there are some recommendations that can really mitigate symptoms associated with menopause. Certainly avoiding trans fats, decreasing saturated fats, and one of the most important things to do is stay plant-strong. That means nutrient dense.

There's this great thing called the ANDI scores—aggregate nutrient density index. For 1 calorie, it's the amount of nutrients. Kale is at the top with 1,000 on the ANDI scale. So if you really want to get the most bang for your buck when it comes to staying nutrient dense, stay plant-strong.

Also, phytoestrogens are really important. Of course, soy comes to mind. There's some controversy around soy, and that's a whole other conversation, but if it's fermented and non-genetically modified, it's a good source of phytoestrogens. It's a plant type of estrogen. Flaxseeds as well. Things like red clover, too.

Bottom Line: In terms of phytoestrogens, a fermented soy product would be miso.

Dr. Lucille: Yes, and I always say fermented is best. So miso, tempeh, natto. Phytoestrogens are different from our own bodies' steroidal estrogens, and they can work as adaptogens—meaning they can block stronger estrogens and, if needed, give a little bit of estrogenic life support.

Bottom Line: So that'll help to replace some of the estrogen that the body's losing at that point in time.

Dr. Lucille: It'll definitely help. This period can happen very quickly for some folks, and depending on the health of the entire endocrine web—you touch one strand and the whole web trembles—it can be a turbulent time. So it will definitely ease the ride, let's say.

Bottom Line: How about some of the chronic inflamers that we all consume in terms of the white breads, the candies, the sugars, the fried foods, the alcohol, and caffeine?

Dr. Lucille: Decreasing those are going to really help mitigate the symptoms associated with menopause, absolutely. Because if you look at it, most of these things are nutritionally valueless. Those nutrients are not just a couple aisles in your health food store; these are what drive your biochemistry.

Every single biochemical reaction you have in your body—the way my finger is going up and down right now, the way my eyes are blinking, my liver is processing the coffee that I drank this morning—they're fueled by co-factors that are vitamins or minerals. And we don't make them; we need to ingest them. So eating those nutritionally valueless foods, to your point, which are very inflammatory, are going to spur on a hot flash. It's also going to increase weight gain. But staying plant-strong and nutrient dense is definitely how you mitigate menopausal symptoms.

Bottom Line: All right, so as painful as it is, the worse your menopausal symptoms are, the more you might really want to watch your diet.

Dr. Lucille: The better your diet needs to be, that's right.

Bottom Line: Or on the flip side of it is, the better your diet, your menopause may not be so bad.

Dr. Lucille: I see it all the time. Someone will come up to me and ask, "What should I take?" I ask her back, "For what?" She says, "For menopause." I ask, "How are you feeling?" "I'm feeling great," she'll say. She's got garlic on her breath and she's got a mustache of green juice!

Bottom Line: Keep eating the kale.

Dr. Lucille: And she really is going through this phase with very, very few symptoms. So you know she doesn't need to do anything. It's all up to each individual's process.

Bottom Line: Interesting. And again, I think a really important point: menopause is not a disease to fear. It's just a phase of evolution.

Dr. Lucille: It is a normal, natural—and guess what?—a once honored, once celebrated time. Hopefully we're going to get our culture turned around and everybody's going to be looking forward to this lovely life phase that all women should experience with pride.

6

Fast Fixes for Stubborn Health Problems

Put Down That Slice of Bread!

What could be more wholesome than whole-wheat bread? For decades, nutritionists and public health experts have almost begged Americans to eat more whole wheat and other grains.

It's bad advice.

Most of us know that white bread is bad for us, but even whole-wheat bread is bad, too. In fact, on the Glycemic Index (GI), which compares the blood sugar effects of carbohydrates, both white bread and whole-wheat bread increase blood glucose more than pure sugar. Aside from some extra fiber, eating two slices of whole-wheat bread is little different from eating a sugary candy bar.

What's particularly troubling is that a high-wheat diet has been linked to obesity, digestive diseases, arthritis, diabetes, dementia and heart disease.

Example: When researchers from the Mayo Clinic and University of Iowa put 215 patients on a wheat-free diet, the obese patients lost an average of nearly 30 pounds in just six months. The patients in the study had celiac disease (a form of wheat sensitivity), but I have seen similar results in nearly everyone who is obese and gives up wheat.

NEW DANGERS FROM A NEW GRAIN

How can a supposedly healthy grain be so bad for you? Because the whole wheat that we eat today has little in common with the truly natural grain. Decades of selective breeding and hybridization by the food industry to increase yield and confer certain baking and aesthetic characteristics on flour have created new proteins in wheat that the human body isn't designed to handle.

William Davis, MD, a preventive cardiologist and medical director of Track Your Plaque, an international heart disease prevention program. Based in Fox Point, Wisconsin, he is author of *Wheat Belly: Lose the Wheat, Lose the Weight, and Find Your Path Back to Health*. Wheatbellyblog.com

The gluten protein in modern wheat is different in structure from the gluten in older forms of wheat. In fact, the structure of modern gluten is something that humans have never before experienced in their 10,000 years of consuming wheat.

Modern wheat also is high in amylo-pectin A, a carbohydrate that is converted to glucose faster than just about any other carbohydrate. I have found it to be a potent appetite stimulant because the rapid rise and fall in blood sugar causes nearly constant feelings of hunger. The gliadin in wheat, another protein, also stimulates the appetite. When people quit eating wheat and are no longer exposed to gliadin and amylopectin A, they typically consume about 400 fewer calories a day.

NOT JUST CELIAC DISEASE

Celiac disease, also known as celiac sprue, is an intense form of wheat sensitivity that damages the small intestine and can lead to chronic diarrhea and cramping, along with impaired absorption of nutrients. But wheat has been linked to dozens of other chronic diseases, including lupus and rheumatoid arthritis. *It also has been linked to…*

• **Insulin resistance and diabetes.** It's not a coincidence that the diabetes epidemic (nearly 26 million Americans have it) parallels the increasing consumption of modern wheat (an average of 134 pounds per person per year) in the US. The surge in blood sugar and insulin that occurs when you eat any kind of wheat eventually causes an increase in visceral (internal) fat. This fat makes the body more resistant to insulin and increases the risk for diabetes.

• **Weaker bones.** A wheat-rich diet shifts the body's chemistry to an acidic (low-pH) state. This condition, known as acidosis, leaches calcium from the bones. Grains—and particularly wheat—account for 38% of the average American's "acid load." This probably is the reason that osteoporosis is virtually universal in older adults.

• **More heart disease.** A diet high in carbohydrates causes an increase in small LDL particles, the type of cholesterol that is most likely to lead to atherosclerosis and cardiovascular diseases. Studies at University of Califor-

nia, Berkeley, found that the concentration of these particles increases dramatically with a high-wheat diet. The increase in small-particle LDL, combined with diabetes and visceral fat, increases the risk for heart disease.

A WHEAT-FREE LIFE

People who crave wheat actually are experiencing an addiction. When the gluten in wheat is digested, it releases molecules known as exorphins, morphinelike compounds that produce mild euphoria. About one-third of people who give up wheat will experience some withdrawal symptoms, including anxiety, moodiness and insomnia. *My advice…*

• **Go cold turkey.** It's the most effective way to break the addiction to wheat. The withdrawal symptoms rarely last more than one week. If you're really suffering, you might want to taper off. Give up wheat at breakfast for a week, and then at breakfast and lunch for another week. Then give it up altogether.

• **Beware of gluten-free products.** People who give up wheat often are tempted to satisfy their craving by buying gluten-free bread or pasta. Don't do it. The manufacturers use substitutes such as brown rice, rice bran, rice starch, corn starch and tapioca starch, which also increase blood glucose and cause insulin surges. Even oatmeal can cause blood sugar to skyrocket.

• **Switch grains.** Small supermarkets now stock quite a few nonwheat grains, such as millet, quinoa, buckwheat and amaranth. They're easy to cook, and they taste good—and they don't have the gluten and other wheat proteins that trigger weight gain, inflammation and insulin resistance.

Helpful: If you aren't willing to give up wheat altogether, you can substitute an older form of wheat, such as spelt or kamut. These grains haven't undergone all of the genetic modifications, so they're somewhat better for you than modern wheat. Any form of wheat can be a problem, however. You'll want to limit yourself to small servings—say, a few ounces once or twice a week.

• **Get plenty of protein.** Protein satisfies the appetite more effectively than carbohydrates. Eat eggs for breakfast and chicken salad for lunch. For dinner, you can have fish or even steak.

New finding: New research has shown that people who eat a reasonable amount of saturated fat in, say, red meat (about 10% or a little more of your total fat calories) have a reduction in small LDL particles, as well as an increase in protective HDL cholesterol.

I'm Kicking the Sugar Habit! Boost Your Immunity, Lose Weight and Feel Better Than You Have in Years

Patricia Farris, MD, FAAD, clinical professor at Tulane University, New Orleans, and member of the media-expert team for the American Academy of Dermatology. She is coauthor, with Brooke Alpert, MS, RD, CDN, of *The Sugar Detox: Lose Weight, Feel Great, and Look Years Younger.*

The average American consumes 32 teaspoons of added sugar per day. That's right—32 teaspoons a day.

We all know that sugar can lead to weight gain, but that's just the beginning. People who eat a lot of sugar have nearly double the risk for heart disease as those who eat less, according to data from the Harvard Nurses' Health Study. They're more likely to develop insulin resistance and diabetes. They also tend to look older because sugar triggers the production of advanced glycation end-products (AGEs), chemical compounds that accelerate skin aging.

If you want to avoid these problems, it's not enough to merely cut back on sugar. In my experience, patients need to eliminate it from their diets—at least at the beginning—just like addicts have to eliminate drugs from their lives. In fact, a study showed that sugar cravings actually are more intense than the cravings for cocaine.

You don't have to give up sugar indefinitely. Once the cravings are gone, you can enjoy sweet foods again—although you probably will be happy consuming far less than before. After a sugar-free "washing out" period, you'll be more sensitive to sweet tastes. You won't want as much.

Bonus: Some people who have completed the four-week diet and stayed on the maintenance program for four or five months lost 35 pounds or more.

FIRST STEP: 3-DAY SUGAR FIX

For sugar lovers, three days without sweet stuff can seem like forever. But it's an essential part of the sugar detox diet because when you go three days without any sugar, your palate readjusts. When you eat an apple after the three-day period, you'll think it's the sweetest thing you've ever tasted. You'll even notice the natural sweetness in a glass of whole or 2% milk (which contains about three teaspoons of naturally occurring sugar).

You may experience withdrawal symptoms during the first three days. These can include fatigue, headache, fogginess and irritability, but soon you'll feel better than you have in years.

Caution: If you have any type of blood sugar problem, including hypoglycemia, insulin resistance or diabetes, you must consult your physician before starting any type of diet, including the sugar detox diet. In addition, if you are on insulin or an oral medication to control blood sugar, it is likely that your dosage will need to be adjusted if you lower your daily sugar intake.

During the three days…

• **No foods or drinks with added sugar.** No candy, cookies, cake, doughnuts, etc.—not even a teaspoon of sugar in your morning coffee.

• **No artificial sweeteners of any kind, including diet soft drinks.** Artificial sweeteners contribute to the sweetness overload that diminishes our ability to taste sugar.

• **No starches.** This includes pasta, cereal, crackers, bread, potatoes and rice.

• **No fruit,** except a little lemon or lime for cooking or to flavor a glass of water or tea. I hesitate to discourage people from eating fruit because it's such a healthy food, but it provides too much sugar when you're detoxing.

87

- **No dairy.** No milk, cream, yogurt or cheese. You can have a little (one to two teaspoons) butter for cooking.
- **Plenty of protein,** including lean red meat, chicken, fish, tofu and eggs.
- **Most vegetables,** such as asparagus, broccoli, cauliflower, celery, peppers, kale, lettuce and more—but no corn, potatoes, sweet potatoes, winter squash, beets or other starchy vegetables.
- **Nuts**—two one-ounce servings a day. Almonds, walnuts, cashews and other nuts are high in protein and fat, both of which will help you feel full. Nuts also will keep your hands (and mouth) busy when you're craving a sugary snack.
- **Lots of water, but no alcohol.** It's a carbohydrate that contains more sugar than you might think. You can drink alcohol later (see below).

NEXT STEP: A FOUR-WEEK PLAN

This is the fun part. During the three-day sugar "fix," you focused on not eating certain foods. Now you'll spend a month adding tasty but nutritious foods back into your diet. You'll continue to avoid overly sweet foods—and you'll use no added sugar—but you can begin eating whole grains, dairy and fresh fruits.

Week 1: **Wine and cheese.** You'll continue to eat healthy foods, but you now can add one apple a day and one daily serving of dairy, in addition to having a splash of milk or cream in your coffee or tea if you like. A serving of dairy could consist of one ounce of cheese…five ounces of plain yogurt…or one-half cup of cottage cheese. You also can have one serving a day of high-fiber crackers, such as Finn Crisp Hi-Fibre or Triscuit Whole Grain Crackers.

You also can start drinking red wine if you wish—up to three four-ounce servings during the first week. Other alcoholic beverages such as white wine, beer and liquor should be avoided. Red wine is allowed because it is high in resveratrol and other antioxidants.

Week 2: **More dairy, plus fruit.** This is when you really start adding natural sugar back into your diet. You can have two servings of dairy daily if you wish and one serving of fruit in addition to an apple a day. You can

have one-half cup of blackberries, blueberries, cantaloupe, raspberries or strawberries each day. Or you can have a grapefruit half. You'll be surprised how sweet fruit really is. You also are allowed one small sweet potato or yam (one-half cup cubed) daily.

Weeks 3 and 4: **Whole grains and more.** The third and fourth weeks are very satisfying because you can start eating grains again. But make sure it's whole grain. Carbohydrates such as white bread, white pasta and white rice are stripped of their fiber during processing, so they are easily broken down into sugar. Whole grains are high in fiber and nutrients and won't give the sugar kick that you would get from processed grains.

Examples: A daily serving of barley, buckwheat, oatmeal (not instant), quinoa, whole-grain pasta, whole-wheat bread or brown rice.

You might find yourself craving something that's deliciously sweet. Indulge yourself with a small daily serving (one ounce) of dark chocolate.

More from Patricia Farris, MD, FAAD…

Test Your Sugar IQ

1. **Which one contains the most sugar?**
   A. Snapple Lemon Tea (16-ounce bottle)
   B. Coca Cola (12-ounce can)
   C. Starbucks Vanilla Latte (Tall, 12 fluid ounces)

2. **True or false?** Humans naturally prefer the taste of sugar from birth.

3. **True or false?** Sugar toxicity causes liver damage.

4. **True or false?** Sugar substitutes help control weight gain.

5. **Which of these foods is hiding the most sugar per half-cup serving?**
   A. Tomato sauce
   B. Salsa
   C. Tomato soup

6. **Reduced-fat packaged foods often have…**
   A. Less sugar than the full-fat version
   B. More sugar than the full-fat version
   C. The same amount of sugar as the full-fat version

7. **True or false?** Eating too much sugar causes wrinkles.

8. **True or false?** Natural sugars, such as honey, have less of an effect on the body than refined sugar does.

9. **True or false?** Natural sugars, such as honey, have fewer calories than refined sugar.

10. **True or false?** People with high blood sugar generally look older.

Answers: 1. B, 2. True, 3. True, 4. False, 5. A, 6. B, 7. True, 8. False, 9. False, 10. True.

From *The Sugar Detox: Lose Weight, Feel Great, and Look Years Younger* by Patricia Farris, MD, FAAD, and Brooke Alpert, MS, RD, CDN. Reprinted courtesy of Da Capo Lifelong Books.

Addicted to "Bad" Foods? It's Not Your Fault! How to Stop Craving the Foods That Make You Fat

Mike Dow, PsyD, clinical director of therapeutic and behavioral services at The Body Well integrative medical center in Los Angeles and host and psychotherapist of the TLC series Freaky Eaters. He is a member of the California Psychological Association and the International Society of Eating Disorder Professionals. He is author of *Diet Rehab: 28 Days to Finally Stop Craving the Foods That Make You Fat.* DrMikeDow.com

---

How often have you heard people say that they're addicted to certain foods? They very well might be. Food addictions are just as real as addictions to drugs or alcohol, just not as obvious. The reason that most diets fail is that they don't address the changes in brain chemistry caused by food that can be more powerful than the effects of cocaine.

Last year, the Scripps Research Institute released a groundbreaking study that found that rats given diets of bacon, sausage, chocolate and cheesecake had sharp rises in dopamine and serotonin, neurochemicals that affect the brain's pleasure centers.

Later, when the researchers withheld these foods and tried to put the rats on a nutritious diet, the rats refused to eat, almost to the point of starvation. The rats even chose to endure painful shocks to get the sweet and fatty foods. They were literally addicted—and it took two weeks for their brains to return to normal. Rats addicted to cocaine, on the other hand, recovered normal brain functions in just two days.

Bottom line: An addiction to food can be harder to overcome than drug addiction.

CHEMISTRY AND WEIGHT GAIN

Most people who are overweight don't experience more hunger than anyone else. They eat too much as a form of self-medication, unconsciously trying to balance levels of the two brain chemicals that are disrupted by unhealthy foods…

•**Dopamine** is the neurochemical that produces excitement and other high-energy feelings. When you eat foods that are high in fat, such as red meat, french fries and cheesecake, you experience a surge of dopamine. It feels good, but the "high" is short-lived. As dopamine levels decline, you may feel listless, sad or depressed. The quickest way to offset the negative feelings is to eat more high-fat foods…and the up-and-down cycle continues.

•**Serotonin** is somewhat different, but just as addictive. It's a "calming" neurochemical that promotes feelings of optimism and hope. It's the primary target of most antidepressant medications. People who consume a lot of sugar or carbohydrates made primarily from white flour (pasta, crackers, white bread) or a combination of sugar and white carbs (cookies, cakes, doughnuts) have increases in serotonin that make them feel good. But, as with dopamine, the effects are temporary unless you keep eating these foods.

BREAK THE CYCLE

Traditional diets mainly deal with calorie restriction. They rarely work because they fail to address the addiction that causes people to overeat in the first place. *Important steps…*

•**Know your pitfalls.** These are the thoughts and activities (and foods) that ultimately lower levels of dopamine and/or serotonin and make you crave another "fix."

Examples: A stressful meeting at work that makes you anxious will increase cravings for sugar or carbohydrates (for the serotonin boost). Spending the night alone in front of the television can lead to loneliness that makes you crave both sugar (for the serotonin boost) and fat (for the dopamine).

Just about everyone with a weight problem engages in what's known as emotional eating. When you realize that you're eating ice cream every night because you're lonely or that you're digging into bags of chips or other snacks when you get anxious or frustrated, you'll be less likely to indulge in this behavior.

• **Increase "booster activities."** These are activities that increase and help maintain healthier levels of serotonin and dopamine. You can tailor these activities to increase levels of either one of these substances. *Examples…*

• For more dopamine…Being active and social are the best ways to boost dopamine. Go to a museum or an art opening. Clean the house while listening to loud music that makes you want to dance. Cook a new, healthful dish. Go dancing.

• For more serotonin…Cultivating relationships and being kind help increase serotonin. Ask a coworker how he/she is feeling. Call a friend or loved one just to say "I'm thinking about you." Give someone a compliment. Play with your dog or cat.

• **Detox gradually.** Just as smokers are more likely to successfully quit when they use nicotine patches or gum, you'll find it easier to give up addictive, high-calorie foods when you replace them with healthier foods that also help balance brain chemistry.

Many of the foods that you already know are healthy will increase serotonin and dopamine. *These include…*

• **Whole grains**
• **Beans**
• **Lean meats,** such as chicken and turkey
• **Low-fat dairy,** such as cottage cheese and yogurt
• **Healthy snacks,** such as unsalted nuts, popcorn and fresh fruits.

Important: It takes at least 10 "exposures" to a healthy food before you'll start to crave it in the same way that you once craved unhealthy choices.

• **Identify risk times.** How many times have you sat down in front of the TV with a full bowl of snacks and emptied it by the end of the show—without even being fully aware that you were eating? Most food addicts snack or binge after 6:00 pm, when they are relaxing at home. This is known as mindless eating, and it's a common behavior of food addicts. People often eat mindlessly in the car as well.

Important: Plan other activities during your own high-risk times. If you tend to snack in the evening, use that time for something else, such as straightening the house or calling friends. It also is helpful to have ready-to-go healthy snacks, such as air-popped popcorn or sliced fruit, for quiet nights when you're reading or watching TV.

• **Allow occasional "slips."** We all have special treats that we don't want to give up. For me, it's buttery movie-theater popcorn. For someone else, it might be ice cream or soft drinks.

In my experience with thousands of patients, those who achieve a healthy relationship with food—those who eat when they're hungry or simply to enjoy a particular food, rather than to fulfill emotional needs—can enjoy up to two servings daily of a pitfall food and still maintain a healthy weight.

To be safe: Don't exceed 300 calories per serving. This might be, for example, half a Big Mac or a small order of fries.

It's not weak to occasionally give in to cravings. As long as your life is full of healthy serotonin- and dopamine-boosting foods and activities, you'll have these cravings only occasionally.

The 30-Second Stress-Busting, Food-Craving Cure

Study titled "Effects of simple distraction tasks on self-induced food cravings in men and women with grade 3 obesity" presented at the Obesity Week 2014 annual meeting of The Obesity Society. Dawn Jackson Blatner, RDN, a registered dietitian nutritionist, certified specialist in sports dietetics and nutrition consultant for the Chicago Cubs, based in Chicago, and author of *The Flexitarian Diet.*

D id your stressful day give you the munchies? Or late-night cravings? It can be tough to resist overeating between meals when mouthwatering images are so intense in your mind.

The quick and easy solution is at your fingertips…

What to do: Tap your head! With either index finger, tap your forehead for 30 seconds.

What it does: This simple motion will reduce the intensity of your food cravings. In a study of 55 obese people at Mount Sinai-St. Luke's Weight Loss Program in New York City, it was the most successful "distraction" tactic…better than tapping your toes, tapping your ear or staring at a blank wall (the control group). All worked, but forehead tapping was the most effective.

How it works: No one knows for sure. But it's possible that simply distracting yourself can be a brief time-out that lets your emotional urges calm down…plus, forehead tapping might stimulate an acupressure region that reduces stress hormone levels.

6 Hot and Healthy Spices to Eat, Inhale, Even Rub

James A. Duke, PhD, an ethnobotanist retired from the USDA, where he developed a database on the health benefits of various plants. He is author of numerous books including *The Green Pharmacy Guide to Healing Foods: Proven Natural Remedies to Treat and Prevent More Than 80 Common Health Concerns.* GreenPharmacy.com

No doubt you've heard about the current "it" spice, turmeric, which shows promise at protecting against cancer, inflammation and Alzheimer's disease. But your spice rack can do so much more for you if you also boost your use of six particular hot and healthy spices.

Naturally, adding these six spices to your food is key—but you also can get some surprising health benefits from inhaling a certain spice-infused steam…and even by rubbing a particular spiced-up sauce on your skin!

According to James A. Duke, PhD, author of *The Green Pharmacy Guide to Healing Food,*

each of the following spices helps improve cholesterol levels, and each has additional benefits as well. *Today's hottest health-boosting spices include…*

•**Black pepper.** Dr. Duke calls piperine, a compound in black pepper, a "potentiator" because it helps our bodies to better absorb and make use of other beneficial herbs and spices. For example, when used together with turmeric, black pepper increases turmeric's protective effects against cancer, inflammation and Alzheimer's disease, Dr. Duke said. Piperine also blocks the formation of new fat cells and aids digestion by increasing the flow of digestive juices.

To up your intake: Add black pepper to just about any savory dish—eggs, soups, sauces, legumes, salads, etc. Note that there is a huge difference in taste between most preground pepper, which is rather bland, and the black pepper that you grind right onto your food from peppercorns. So get yourself a pepper mill…and also, for maximum potency, chose the most pungent peppercorns you can find.

•**Cardamom.** Used as an aphrodisiac in Middle Eastern countries, both the pods and the seeds within help stimulate the central nervous system. "Cardamom is the richest source I know of the compound cineole, which helps improve memory by preventing the breakdown of the neurotransmitter acetylcholine," Dr. Duke said. Cardamom also contains chemicals that ease stomach and intestinal spasms, reduce gas and speed the movement of food through the digestive tract.

Breathe it in: We absorb cineole best by inhaling it, Dr. Duke noted, so add one or two cardamom pods or a bit of ground cardamom to a cup of hot water, then inhale the steam for several minutes. (Do not inhale ground cardamom directly, as this could irritate the lungs.)

Add to food: Try ground cardamom seeds in rice pilaf and meat dishes.

Caution: If you have gallstones, do not go overboard on cardamom—excessive amounts (beyond what is typically used in food) could exacerbate gallstone-related pain.

•**Fennel seeds.** If you've eaten in an Indian restaurant, you've probably seen a bowl of small seeds (some candied, some not) where you'd normally find after-dinner mints. Those are fennel seeds, and they're there for good reason—with an aroma reminiscent of licorice, the seeds are an effective breath freshener. Fennel seeds also are a digestive aid, relaxing the smooth muscles that line the digestive tract and relieving flatulence, bloating and gas. They soothe the tough-to-relieve symptoms of inflammatory bowel disease.

Try it: Chew whole fennel seeds to freshen your breath...use ground fennel seeds to add flavor to spice rubs for meat or fish, or sprinkle it into vegetable dishes. For best flavor, grind your own seeds using a small coffee grinder or a pestle and mortar, or place the seeds in a sealed bag and crush them with a rolling pin.

•**Fenugreek seeds.** Many women first learn about fenugreek while nursing their infants because the spice stimulates the production of breast milk. It also is an anti-inflammatory...and it helps stabilize blood glucose in people with diabetes by slowing absorption of sugars. Fenugreek's flavor is a cross between maple sugar and celery, though it can be bitter if used in excess. If you can't find it in your supermarket, look instead in Indian or Middle Eastern groceries (where it may be called methi) or purchase it online.

Cooking tip: Fenugreek adds a distinctive flavor to soups, stews and sauces. The seeds are hard, though, so you may want to buy them preground or use a small coffee grinder...or dry-fry the whole seeds in a skillet over medium heat for several minutes before adding them to whatever you're cooking.

•**Horseradish.** This pungent root—which lends a distinctive sharp flavor to cocktail sauce (or Bloody Mary cocktails)—is loaded with *isothiocyanates*. These compounds have antiseptic properties and also may help protect against the development of certain cancers by promoting elimination of carcinogens from the body.

Healthful flavor boost: Add ground horseradish to dips, hummus, mustard and other condiments, or spread it on a sandwich.

Aromatherapy for colds: Next time you have a cold, try grating some fresh horseradish and inhaling the aroma to open your sinuses and kill germs. Start by inhaling gently—fresh horseradish can be strong, and you don't want to give yourself an uncomfortable blast.

•**Red pepper.** Chile peppers—from which paprika, cayenne pepper, red pepper flakes, and Tabasco sauce and similar hot sauces derive—contain the super-spicy compound capsaicin. This is a potent antioxidant that helps neutralize cell-damaging free radicals. Capsaicin also curbs the appetite...raises body temperature...and may help kill off cancer cells. In addition, capsaicin is used as a topical pain reliever, neutralizing the nerves so they are less sensitive.

Topical treatment: To ease his own knee pain, Dr. Duke has been rubbing on a few drops of hot sauce from the grocery store, as often as needed. He has been using this remedy for several years and it's working for him, but he noted that, for some people, the treatment seems to stop helping after awhile. (If you try this, use your palm rather than fingertips, then wash hands thoroughly so you won't inadvertently get any of the stinging sauce into a cut or your eyes or onto any mucous membrane.) Another option is to use a nonprescription capsaicin cream, such as Zostrix.

Add zip to foods: Add a dash of any red pepper product to pasta sauces, casseroles and veggie dishes...or even sprinkle a bit on ice cream!

How much to use? With any of these spices, the effective (and palate-pleasing) dosage can vary greatly from one person to the next. Dr. Duke recommends starting conservatively, with just a small amount. He said, "If you don't enjoy the flavor, you're using too much. If you like the way you feel, you're probably getting a good dose."

Neroli Oil Soothes Menopausal Symptoms

Study titled "Effects of Inhalation of Essential Oil of Citrus aurantium L. var. amara on Menopausal Symptoms, Stress, and Estrogen in Postmenopausal Women: A Randomized Controlled Trail," published in *Evidence-Based Complementary and Alternative Medicine.*

Are menopausal symptoms—the hot flashes, night sweats, insomnia and moodiness among all else—cramping your style...stressing your relationships...in short, ruining your life? Sure, hormone replacement therapy (HRT) is an option, but maybe its risks, such as blood clots, gallstones, breast cancer and stroke, have nixed that idea for you.

There's another great way that's helping women wind down and recharge...and stop hot flashes.

No, it's not another supplement, mind trick or exercise routine. It's aromatherapy using a lusciously exotic scent—neroli oil.

SNIFF TEST

Neroli oil is extracted from the blossoms of the bitter orange tree and is rich in *limonene*, a compound that has antianxiety and muscle-relaxing effects. Neroli oil vapor, when inhaled, is known to relieve anxiety, stress and depression, reduce high blood pressure and stimulate an underactive libido. Because symptoms such as mood swings and underactive libido are so common in menopause, a group of Korean researchers decided to scientifically test whether neroli oil had an effect on those and other menopausal symptoms.

Here's what they did. The team recruited 63 healthy menopausal women and divided them into three groups. One group received several vials of a 0.1% concentration of neroli essential oil in scentless sweet almond oil...the other, a 0.5% concentration (in scentless sweet almond oil)...and the third group received plain scentless sweet almond oil (a placebo).

The women sat in a comfortable position every morning and evening for five days and inhaled the oil vapor for five minutes at each sitting. To inhale the scent, the women simply poured a small vial of oil on a fragrance pad and held the pad about 12 inches from their noses while they breathed normally.

Before and after the five-day treatment period, each woman was given special questionnaires that rated and scored their quality of life and levels of stress and sexual desire. Blood pressure and pulse were also checked, and blood tests were done to measure cortisol (a stress hormone) and estrogen levels.

The results: Compared with the placebo group, women inhaling neroli felt better and had fewer hot flashes. After the five days of daily aromatherapy, their quality-of-life scores improved by an average of 28% in the women smelling 0.1% neroli oil and 20% in the women smelling 0.5% neroli oil compared with an average 7% improvement in women smelling the placebo oil.

Sexual desire also got a lift in the women who inhaled neroli oil, most especially if they were inhaling the 0.5% concentration. It improved by an average 113% in women using the higher concentration and 27% in women using the 0.1% concentration. Meanwhile, sexual desire took a 50% dive in women using the placebo oil.

HOW TO BENEFIT FROM NEROLI OIL

Some pure essential oils, such as clove and cinnamon, come with strong precautions because they can irritate the skin or lungs. Neroli oil is much milder. Still, no undiluted essential oil should be daubed on the skin straight out of the bottle—remember, this is concentrated stuff. A few drops should be placed in a scentless "carrier oil," such as sweet almond oil or jojoba oil.

To approximate your own 0.5% concentration of neroli oil, the ratio should be four drops of the essential oil per ounce of carrier oil. (A good aromatherapy oil will come with its own dropper.)

Don't want to fuss with mixing essential oils and carriers? Another simple way to enjoy aromatherapy is to place up to five drops of an essential oil in a pot of hot water and, keeping a safe distance of about a foot away, breathe the steam. Or consider purchasing an aromatherapy diffuser and vaporizer. They come in different styles and have different user directions that come with the packaging. These gadgets either warm an essential oil or mix it with steam to create a scented vapor. They cost anywhere from a few bucks to about $60 and can be easily found in department stores or online through Amazon.com and other sellers.

No side effects were seen in the study, so why not take a few minutes a day to stop and smell the neroli to manage The Change?

Nosebleed Know-How

To stop a nosebleed, sit upright, lean forward and pinch the soft part of your nose with your thumb and forefinger for five to 15 minutes.

To prevent recurrent nosebleeds: Humidify your living space…lubricate your nose with saline spray or a thin film of petroleum jelly. Also, talk to your doctor—the blood vessel causing nosebleeds may need to be cauterized.

Caution: If a nosebleed doesn't stop after 30 minutes, go to the hospital. A doctor may have to insert packing material into the nostril or surgery may be needed.

Mayo Clinic Health Letter, 200 First St. SW, Rochester, Minnesota 55905, http://healthletter.mayoclinic.com.

How to Stop Yourself from Throwing Up

Deborah Serani, PsyD, a psychologist in private practice in Smithtown, New York, and author of *Living with Depression.* DrDeborahSerani.com

If you get queasy easily, take a deep breath before you read this.

Do you remember the scene in the movie *Stand By Me* in which one pie-eating contestant vomits and that triggers all the others to "lose their lunch," so to speak?

That may have been funny to watch, but it's not so funny when you're the one in a room

(or, worse, in a vehicle) with someone who starts in with those telltale gagging sounds.

As your neighbor gets sick and you see and smell the vomit, you start feeling nauseated and sweaty and may even join in by vomiting, too.

It's a fact—vomiting is contagious. But there are ways to keep yourself out of it—simple things that you can do instantly, the moment you feel it coming on.

EMPATHY IN OVERDRIVE

Why do we often get nauseated when we see someone else vomit? We're wired to mirror the feelings of people around us. It's a leftover reflex that protected us from sickness back when we were cavemen and cavewomen. The reaction was a way of having early humans purge their stomach contents if they saw someone else (who likely ate the same food) become sick. Expelling it quickly would help them recover sooner.

The same mechanism (technically called "mirror neuron system") explains why we scratch our scalps when we hear of someone else being infected with lice. In fact, brain scans have shown that the parts of the brain that are activated when we smell something foul or prick our finger are also activated when we watch a video of other people smelling something foul or having their fingers pricked.

Social scientists call it emotional contagion. It's a form of empathy—but in this case, it's related not to helping other people but to protecting ourselves.

STOP THAT ICK!

You can, though, counteract the sensations that you feel when witnessing someone else get sick. The first and obvious step would be to remove yourself from the situation, but if you can't physically get away, try to engage all of your senses to redirect your mind and, in effect, override the reflex. This will put some emotional distance between you and the sick scene.

WHAT TO DO IMMEDIATELY…

• **Use your nose.** Going outside to inhale fresh air or opening a window would be best, but when you can't do that, sniff the inside of your wrist or wherever you tend to spray cologne or perfume. This way, you may not smell the vomit! If you're very prone to nausea, consider keeping a portable scent in your pocket or purse at all times—such as a little bag of cloves…a small box of potpourri…or a tiny bottle of an essential oil such as peppermint, lavender or lemon. If you don't wear cologne or perfume or don't want to carry anything around, at the very least, quickly place your hands over your nose and mouth and inhale whatever scent is on them, such as soap residue from the last time you washed them.

• **Speak up.** Repeat to yourself (either aloud or silently), "I am OK. I am not going to get sick." This may sound silly, but these types of affirmations can positively impact your state of mind.

• **Reach out and touch something.** Get some tactile sensations going that cause a little—not a lot—of pain. For example, try pinching your arm slightly…tapping your fist onto your thigh…tugging on a few strands of hair…digging your nails gently into your arm…or biting your lower lip.

• **Try acupressure.** Pressing the inner parts of both of your wrists together may help lessen nausea.

IF THE SMELL LINGERS…

• **Suck on candy or chew gum.** Having a pleasant taste in your mouth might distract you. Peppermint, especially, is known to be soothing to the stomach, so it may help to keep some peppermint-flavored gum or mints in your bag at all times. (If you suffer from reflux, choose a different flavor because you may find peppermint to be irritating.)

• **Distract your eyes and ears.** Picture yourself in a pleasant situation—perhaps you might envision yourself lying on a beach in Hawaii…or singing a song on a Broadway stage…or hitting the winning three-pointer in a basketball game. Or just look away and turn your attention to something else (besides the vomiting) that's going on in the room—for example, focus on a painting or whatever is on TV. Or look around in your purse or briefcase for something that can grab your attention for a few minutes—for instance, play a game on your smartphone or listen to a song that you love on your portable music player.

Remember, with contagious nausea, it's your mind that is making you feel sick…and your mind that can take that feeling away.

Alternative Toenail Fungus Treatment

Applying a mentholated ointment such as Vicks VapoRub onto infected toenails daily has been found to help cure or partially clear up the fungus as effectively as over-the-counter fungus products such as Lamisil or Lotrimin. The ingredients in mentholated ointments (thymol, menthol, camphor and oil of eucalyptus) have been shown to be effective in decreasing fungus in lab experiments.

Best: Before applying mentholated ointment, wipe affected nails with a cotton ball soaked in white vinegar. Vinegar is acidic, and acid decreases the pH of the area, which helps to retard fungal growth.

Sally Stroud, EdD, associate professor, college of nursing, Medical University of South Carolina, Charleston.

Quick Cure for Bad Breath

For unpleasant breath odor, take liquid chlorophyll after meals. The antioxidants in chlorophyll, found in the green pigment of plants, have deodorizing properties that neutralize the gases that rise from the stomach and intestines and from bacteria in the mouth. Liquid chlorophyll is available at health-food stores. Follow label instructions. Consult a physician if you have chronic bad breath. In rare cases, it is a sign of kidney or liver problems.

Mark A. Stengler, NMD, naturopathic medical doctor and founder and medical director of the Stengler Center for Integrative Medicine, Encinitas, California. He is the author of many books, including *The Natural Physician's Healing Therapies* and coauthor of *Prescription for Natural Cures* and *Prescription for Drug Alternatives*.

Don't Let Them Tell You Gluten Intolerance Isn't Real

Study titled "Small Amounts of Gluten in Subjects with Suspected Nonceliac Gluten Sensitivity—a Randomized, Double-Blind, Placebo-Controlled, Cross-Over Trial," by researchers in the department of internal medicine at University of Pavia, and the department of medical and surgical sciences at University of Bologna, both in Italy, published in *Clinical Gastroenterology and Hepatology*.

You may have been told that unless you have the autoimmune disorder celiac disease, you're not gluten intolerant, and the pain and bloating you blame on sensitivity to gluten is all in your head. Meanwhile, the gluten-free food industry is booming as never before, and many people are singing the benefits of a gluten-free life. So…is gluten sensitivity real? Or is it just the latest craze?

GLUTEN SENSITIVITY IS REAL—BUT NOT ALWAYS

According to a new study, it is entirely possible to be sensitive to gluten without having a wheat allergy or celiac disease. But it's also possible that gluten exerts a nocebo effect on some folks. A nocebo effect is an ill effect caused by the suggestion or belief that something—in this case gluten/wheat–is harmful.

The study, conducted by researchers from the Universities of Pavia and Bologna in Italy, involved 59 participants who had self-described gluten intolerance. They reported symptoms such as bloating, gassiness, diarrhea, headache and brain fog. Before starting the study, all of the participants had blood work and biopsies of the small intestine to rule out wheat allergies and celiac disease.

To identify whether gluten was actually causing symptoms, the researchers put participants on a strict gluten-free diet for five weeks, and during part of that time had them take one of two daily pills—either wheat gluten or a placebo. Participants switched off during the study so that everyone had a chance to take gluten pills and placebos during different weeks (but without knowing which was which, of course). Each gluten pill contained

about the amount of gluten found in two slices of white bread.

Participants completed daily questionnaires that measured the severity of a wide range of symptoms on a scale of zero (not affected) to three (severely affected). In addition to intestinal symptoms, such as pain, bloating and gas, nonintestinal symptoms frequently associated with gluten intolerance, such as headache, tiredness, malaise, brain fog and anxiety, were also asked about.

The results: The participants' total average symptom severity score was 30% higher during the week they were given gluten compared with the week they received placebo pills, showing that gluten did make a difference for some. However, when the researchers plotted each participant's weekly scores on grids to view correlations between how each person felt during gluten and gluten-free weeks, they found that about half of the participants complained about symptoms to the same degree whether they were receiving gluten or not. The remaining participants either logged in more symptoms when they were receiving gluten or placebo. Of the nine patients who recorded more symptoms while on gluten than placebo, three (amounting to 5% of the study group) had scores that consistently showed symptom flares when exposed to gluten but not placebo. Symptoms of bloating, abdominal pain, brain fog, depression and canker sores—the most common intestinal and nonintestinal symptoms experienced across the board—were consistently and significantly worse during the week of gluten exposure in these patients compared with the rest of the study group. The researchers commented that these participants likely had true gluten intolerance despite lack of wheat allergy or celiac disease and that the other six participants may have had a lesser level of gluten sensitivity. They also point out that the dose of gluten given was low, and so higher amounts might have shown greater sensitivity in more of the participants.

DO YOU REALLY NEED TO BE GLUTEN-FREE?

These study findings add weight to both sides of the argument…yes, gluten intolerance does seem to occur in a small percentage of people. On the other hand, gluten may not actually be behind symptoms that many people experience and attribute to gluten intolerance.

If you notice that you have abdominal pain or bloating, fogginess or low mood after eating foods with gluten, you can test whether you are truly sensitive to it by going gluten-free for one or two weeks, evaluating whether symptoms improve and then reintroducing bread or pasta back into your diet and again evaluating symptoms. A better strategy, though, would be to consult a dietitian or naturopathic doctor who can expertly evaluate your symptoms and guide you through a diet regimen to correct the problem without compromising nutrition—whether that means avoiding gluten or following some other strategy.

What's Really Causing Your Gas and Bloating?

Douglas A. Drossman, MD, codirector emeritus at the University of North Carolina Center for Functional GI and Motility Disorders and professor emeritus of medicine and psychiatry at the University of North Carolina School of Medicine in Chapel Hill. He is also the president of the Rome Foundation, an international nonprofit group that develops guidelines for the diagnosis and treatment of functional GI disorders.

Ugh! Here comes another gas attack. Or maybe it's bloating that's got you feeling so out of sorts. If you're lucky, you can avoid gas and/or bloating by forgoing the usual triggers—carbonated drinks…some high-fiber foods such as beans…chewing gum…and artificial sweeteners and the fruit sugar fructose.

But sometimes the source of this all-too-common gastrointestinal (GI) discomfort isn't so obvious. If your symptoms don't ease within a few weeks…or they have no apparent reason and tend to come and go, you and your doctor may need to do some investigating. *The following health problems can cause gas and/ or bloating but often go undetected—especially in the early stages…*

• **Aerophagia (air swallowing).** Swallowing too much air can stretch the stomach and cause bloating. This often occurs when people are experiencing anxiety or can even become an unconscious habit. It can also happen when chewing gum, using a straw or drinking carbonated beverages.

What to do: Consider stress-reducing activities like deep breathing, meditation or yoga. If symptoms are severe, see a counselor for stress-management techniques.

• **Irritable bowel syndrome (IBS).** As many as one in five adults experiences the chronic symptoms of IBS—abdominal pain, bloating, gas, diarrhea and/or constipation—to some degree. IBS can have many causes, but typically nerves in the GI tract are extremely sensitive to food and gas passing through the bowel, triggering discomfort.

What to do: An IBS diagnosis includes regular abdominal pain that is relieved by a bowel movement, along with symptoms of bloating, diarrhea and/or constipation.

If you have IBS, your doctor may prescribe antispasmodics, such as *dicyclomine* (Bentyl) and *hyoscyamine* (Levsin), that may help relieve your symptoms. Since stress can trigger IBS symptoms, try to manage it with yoga, massage, meditation and counseling, if needed.

• **Functional dyspepsia.** After eating, the stomach in a healthy adult can expand in volume up to four times its normal size. But with functional dyspepsia, the muscles don't relax properly and the stomach remains small, leaving you feeling full and bloated after just a few bites.

What to do: If symptoms are stress-related, relaxation techniques, such as deep breathing or biofeedback, may be effective. An antianxiety drug, such as buspirone (BuSpar), can also help because it helps to relax the stomach.

• **Celiac disease.** People with celiac disease are sensitive to gluten, a protein in wheat, barley and rye that can produce inflammation in the bowel, resulting in bloating, gas, abdominal cramps and diarrhea.

What to do: If you suffer from the digestive symptoms described above—especially if you also have any nutritional deficiencies and/or experience frequent fatigue—see your doctor. Celiac disease is diagnosed with a blood test followed by an endoscopic biopsy. By avoiding foods and products that contain gluten, most sufferers can eliminate symptoms. For a list of hidden sources of gluten, go to Celiac.org.

More serious but less common causes of gas and/or bloating...

•**Diverticulitis.** This condition occurs when small pouches in the walls of the colon become inflamed and/or infected—often due to small tears caused by stool trapped in the pouches. It not only causes gas and bloating but also pain in the lower left side of the pelvis, where pouches get infected.

What to do: If you're having severe abdominal pain with fever and vomiting, see your doctor right away—you could have a serious infection that requires antibiotics and possibly emergency surgery. Sometimes, however, diverticulitis is mild, and symptoms may improve if you apply heat to the painful area...go on a liquid diet—including clear broth, clear fruit juice (such as apple), gelatin and plain tea—for a few days to "rest" your digestive system...and/or take antibiotics if needed to treat an infection.

•**Gallstones.** They often cause no symptoms, but if gallstones block the duct where the gallbladder empties, the gallbladder stretches, resulting in distension and pain, as well as bloating and gas.

What to do: If you suffer bloating and gas, pain in the upper-right abdomen (where the gallbladder is located), nausea and fever, see your doctor. He/she will perform an ultrasound to check for gallstones. Gallstone removal, which is routinely performed via laparoscopic surgery or, in some cases, endoscopy, is often recommended.

•**Certain cancers.** With advanced colorectal cancer, the bowel can become blocked, which leads to gas, bloating and blood in the stool. Ovarian cancer often causes subtle symptoms that may include bloating and feeling full quickly.

What to do: With colorectal cancer, regular colonoscopies after age 50 (or after age 40 if a close family member has had the disease) will catch suspicious polyps before a malignancy develops. Women who experience the symptoms described above for more than two or three weeks—especially if they are accompanied by

pelvic pain and/or an urgent or frequent need to urinate—should see a gynecologist.

QUICK RELIEF

If your gas and/or bloating is only occasional, consider trying...

•**Probiotics, which promote the growth of "good" bacteria in the bowel.** One study found that Lactobacillus acidophilus and Bifidobacterium lactis helped bloating by replacing the bad (gas-causing) bacteria with good (gas-relieving) bacteria in people with bowel disorders, such as IBS or functional dyspepsia. In another study, probiotics were found to relieve intestinal gas.

What to do: Try a daily probiotic in supplement form or via probiotic-rich fermented foods and beverages such as kefir, miso or kimchi.

Easy DIY Test for Strep

Andrew M. Fine, MD, MPH, attending physician, emergency medicine, Boston Children's Hospital, assistant professor of pediatrics, Harvard Medical School. His study was published in *Annals of Internal Medicine*.

Your throat hurts so much that you just want to stay curled up on the couch. But you're worried that a strep infection might be to blame, so you drag yourself to the doctor's office. Wouldn't it be nice if there were a test you could take yourself to rule out strep—without having to leave the comfort of home?

Well, according to a new study, there is a self-test that can determine with a good degree of accuracy whether or not a sore throat is likely to be from strep. And you don't need a swab or any apparatus, in fact. *All you need to do is ask yourself two simple questions...*

THE TWO KEYS

Sore throats lead to 12 million visits to the doctor's office, health clinic or emergency room in the US each year. Only about 10% of sore throats in adults (and about 25% in children) are due to the group A Streptococcus bacterium. A definitive diagnosis of strep requires swabbing the throat and then running a test (a throat culture or DNA probe). When a strep test is positive, antibiotics generally are warranted because untreated strep can lead to rheumatic fever, scarlet fever, heart damage and/or kidney damage. However, the vast majority of sore throats are due to common viruses that won't respond to antibiotics. Why not give antibiotics just in case without bothering to test for strep? Because the drugs can cause side effects such as severe diarrhea…and overuse contributes to antibiotic resistance.

Researchers wanted to explore whether there was a way that regular people, at home, could determine whether they were at very low risk for strep and thus could safely wait to see whether their symptoms would clear up on their own. For the study, the researchers used data provided by CVS, the drugstore chain that operates MinuteClinics. Everyone who visited a MinuteClinic complaining of a sore throat was given a rapid strep test and also questioned about symptoms. Over the course of two years in nine markets around the country, there were 71,766 visits by sore throat patients age 15 or older…24% of those ended up testing positive for strep.

When doctors check for strep, they look for swollen lymph nodes in the neck plus fluid or pus around the tonsils. But patients generally cannot check for such signs themselves. Because the aim of this study was to explore a do-it-yourself system that patients could use, the researchers focused on patients' reports of symptoms that could be assessed without a physical exam—such as fever, cough, headache, earache, stomachache, nausea, difficulty sleeping, etc.

After analyzing all the symptom reports and strep test results, the researchers determined that just two questions—*Have you had a fever in the last 24 hours?*…and *Do you have a cough?*—generally were sufficient to determine whether the likelihood of strep was low enough that a person could skip the doctor visit and strep test.

Explanation: Strep usually is accompanied by fever, whereas a cough usually indicates a virus.

WHEN STREP IS GOING AROUND

There was actually more to this study, because the researchers also factored in the "local recent incidence of strep," meaning the percentage of strep tests done within a given region during the previous 14 days that turned out to have positive results. By combining information about local strep outbreaks with the fever/cough clues, it was possible to predict even more accurately whether a given patient did or did not have strep.

Someday soon, a smartphone app or website might provide the public with that kind of local outbreak information by Zip code. In the meantime, you can get a sense of this simply by phoning your doctor's office and asking whether strep is "going around" in your area.

Bottom line: If you have a sore throat, you should get tested for strep if you have or recently had a fever and you do not have a cough—particularly if your doctor tells you that he's been seeing a lot of strep lately…or if you are the type of person who prefers to err on the side of caution.

But you may want to wait a few days if you have not had a fever or if you have been coughing—especially if your doctor says that there's no current strep outbreak in your area—to see if the sore throat clears up on its own, as viruses generally do.

Caveat: These guidelines are intended for adults. Children who have sore throats, with or without a fever or cough, generally should see their doctors to get tested for strep because the infection is more common among kids. And even in adults, these guidelines are not foolproof—so if your symptoms worsen, do get yourself to the doctor and get tested for strep.

7

Color Away Your Anxiety and Stress

The Latest Anti-Stress Trend: Coloring Books for Adults

Heard about the new relaxation trend? You don't need a yoga mat or soothing scents or a Tibetan drum. You just need a box of Crayolas or colored pencils and a coloring book for grown-ups.

That's right. It's good-bye *SpongeBob*...hello *Secret Garden* and *Enchanted Forest*. These beautifully detailed black-and-white drawings of plants, flowers, trees, animals and birds by UK illustrator Johanna Basford are topping best-seller lists.

It's a full-blown trend. There's *Adult Coloring Book: Stress Relieving Patterns*, *Color Me Calm: 100 Coloring Templates for Meditation and Relaxation* and *The Mindfulness Colouring Book: Anti-Stress Art Therapy for Busy People*. You can find adult coloring book series from the publishers Creative Haven and Skyhorse Publishing. Even Marvel, the comic book and movie giant, has released an *Age of Ultron* coloring book (based on the company's blockbuster *Avengers* series) for adults, followed by *Little Marvel by Skottie Young Coloring Book* (featuring line art of award-winning illustrator and cartoonist Skottie Young's comic book covers and interior pages) and *Civil War Coloring Book* (with iconic superheroes Captain American and Iron Man) in early 2016. What should we make of this newest publishing phenomenon? Is coloring for grown-ups an affordable, effective therapeutic pastime that reduces health-sapping stress? A cool new way to release your inner child? Or just a fad with no real health benefits?

HONEST-TO-GOODNESS MEDITATION...WITH CRAYONS

Let's cut to the chase. While no health studies have specifically examined coloring books for adults, the approach makes sense.

Coloring combines creative and aesthetic elements with fine motor skills, and that engages

Allen Elkin, PhD, clinical psychologist, director, Stress Management and Counseling Center, New York City, and author of *Stress Management for Dummies*.

different parts of your brain in ways that can be relaxing and satisfying and can enhance your attention. Just as with knitting, coloring can be distracting in a way that gets you away from your worries and neurotic thinking—and that can be very therapeutic. Like meditation, coloring is a mindful activity that can help you focus. It distracts you, but just enough.

Having a creative hobby like coloring might even enhance your performance at work. In a pair of studies published in *Journal of Occupational and Organizational Psychology*, researchers from San Francisco State University examined the relationships between nonwork creative activities (such as doing art or crafts, writing poetry, playing music and the like) and performance-related behaviors at work. They found that people who engaged in creative activities outside work gained a sense of mastery and control and experienced relaxation, which helped relieve their stress. What's more, their colleagues reported that people with these hobbies showed more creativity and more of a team spirit at work.

So go ahead—release your inner artist. Stay in the lines...or be a rebel and color outside them. These are not your elementary school coloring books—they can get pretty intricate and engrossing. Plus, when the crayons or colored pencils are put away, you might even have something worthy of your refrigerator door.

For sample art to color, see pages 117-119.

Tap Away Fears and Phobias

Shoshana Garfield, PhD, is a psychologist, Registered Trauma Specialist and Neurolinguistic Programming Master Practitioner in practice in Uplands, Wales. ShoshanaGarfield.com

Thought Field Therapy (TFT) is a technique designed to help people permanently free themselves from phobias (strong, irrational fears of things that pose little or no actual danger), such as fear of spiders or of public speaking...and even from post-traumatic stress disorder (PTSD), an anxiety disorder that can develop after a terrifying event in which grave harm occurred or was threatened. No medications are used, so there are no side effects. TFT falls within the field of energy psychology and involves thinking about the feared object or event while tapping specific points on the face and body and humming, counting or moving the eyes.

TFT has roots in acupuncture, in that you tap on points that correspond to energy meridians. This helps unblock the body's energy system, which can become overwhelmed by fear. TFT also simultaneously provides sensory data to the right brain (the emotional side) and left brain (the logical side). This stimulates activity of both brain hemispheres and of the corpus callosum that connects them...deactivates signals associated with fear-triggered hyperarousal of the limbic system...and "rewires" cognitive function, releasing distress.

Evidence: In a recent study, PTSD patients treated with TFT showed dramatic decreases in nightmares, flashbacks, concentration problems, jumpiness, aggression and isolation. Other studies have demonstrated TFT's effectiveness in reducing depression...and in patients with anxiety disorder, EEG scans showed that abnormal brain wave patterns associated with anxiety normalized after TFT treatment.

A classic example from TFT founder Roger Callahan, PhD, describes a woman who had a lifelong fear of water. After more than a year of ineffective conventional treatment, Dr. Callahan instructed the woman to tap a spot under each eye while looking at a swimming pool. After a few minutes of tapping, she said that she no longer felt any fear, then ran to the pool and splashed water on her face—something she could not do previously.

TRYING TFT FOR YOURSELF

For best results, work with a psychologist trained in TFT who can provide testimonials from other patients with phobias similar to yours.

Referrals: Association for Comprehensive Energy Psychology (visit *www.energypsych.org* and click on "membership" and then "member directory")...or Association for the Advancement of Meridian Energy Techniques (visit *www.aamet.org* and click on "search members and events")...or Dr. Roger Callahan (*www.*

rogercallahan.com). Results might be seen after just one treatment for a simple phobia or might take nine months or longer for PTSD. Are you skeptical? That's OK—because TFT works even if you don't believe in it.

For simple fears that are not deeply interwoven with complex traumas, you may find relief on your own with the tapping sequence below. Practice it several times until you know the steps...then do the sequence whenever you anticipate or encounter the feared object or event. (Use common sense, of course—for instance, by tapping before you get behind the wheel, rather than while you are driving.) The routine takes just a few minutes and, though it may seem complicated at first, it soon becomes second nature, Dr. Garfield said. *Demo: www.youtube.com/watch?v=ntWUsL5hZJ0.*

STEP 1: **Focus attention on the thing you fear.** For instance, visualize a spider or imagine driving through a construction zone

Important: **Keep thinking about the object of your fear throughout your TFT session.**

STEP 2: **Rate your fear level on a scale of zero to 10.** Zero would indicate no distress whatsoever and 10 would be the worst it could possibly be. Remember this number.

STEP 3: **Tap.** Use the tips of the index and middle fingers of either hand to tap firmly (but not hard enough to hurt) five to 10 times, at a moderately fast pace. First tap four inches below either armpit (about at the center of the band on your bra)...then tap one inch below the center of either eye.

STEP 4: **Perform the nine-step "gamut sequence."** Make a loose fist with your nondominant hand and locate what TFT practitioners call the gamut spot on the back of that hand, in the hollow an inch below the knuckles of the ring and little fingers. Start tapping this gamut spot with the index and middle fingers of your dominant hand.

Continuing tapping, giving five to 10 taps for each of the following actions.

Gamut sequence: Open eyes wide...close eyes...open eyes and (keeping head still) look down and to the left...look down and to the

right...roll eyes around counterclockwise...roll eyes around clockwise...hum a few bars of any song (activating the right brain)...count aloud from one to five (activating the left brain)... hum again. When finished, repeat the gamut sequence a second time.

STEP 5: **Rate your fear again, from zero to 10.** If your score has dropped to zero, terrific! If it has not, repeat all the TFT steps one or more times, continuing to visualize the object of your phobia. Then, again rate your fear level—which may now be much lower.

Crazy with Stress? Craft Your Way to Calm

Nancy Monson is a certified health coach and creativity expert based in Shelton, Connecticut. She is the author of four books, including *Craft to Heal: Soothing Your Soul with Sewing, Painting, and Other Pastimes.* CreativeWellness.us

When my mother was diagnosed with dementia, the challenges of caregiving coupled with the intense emotional strain sent my stress levels skyrocketing. How did I cope? By pulling out my art supplies and making mixed-media collages featuring my mom. The creative outlet calmed frazzled nerves and helped me work through my grief.

I speak not only from personal healing but also from professional experience. As a certified health coach and author of *Craft to Heal: Soothing Your Soul with Sewing, Painting, and Other Pastimes*, I have done extensive research on the psychological and physical health benefits—including stress reduction—of creative hobbies. For instance, a classic study, cited in *The Journal of the American Medical Association*, found that women who sew experience a significant drop in heart rate and blood pressure, perhaps because such creative pursuits allow the body to rest from the pressures of everyday life.

In other words, the magic of crafts is that they distract you from your worries and let you focus on the simple joys of the here and now. But to reap the benefits, you need to approach your creative activities the right way.

Otherwise, crafts can become a source of annoyance, ratcheting up rather than relieving stress. *Helpful*...

• **Give yourself permission to craft.** Many women feel that they're being too self-indulgent if they take time to pursue a hobby when they "should" be working, cleaning or caretaking. So instead of "shoulding" all over yourself, reframe your inner dialog—reminding yourself that your craft is like an essential vitamin that supports your health and well-being.

• **Pursue crafts that suit your personality.** Are you a detail-oriented, organized person? You'll get great satisfaction from activities that require precision and planning, such as quilting, beadwork, decorative painting, mosaic, embroidery or woodworking. If you're a spontaneous, embrace-the-chaos kind of woman, give yourself some messy good times—for instance, with pottery, abstract painting, fabric dyeing, collage or gardening.

Best: If an activity feels tedious or frustrating, drop it and try something else...keep experimenting until you've discovered several hobbies that you truly enjoy.

• **Choose the right activity at the right time.** Having a repertory of different crafts allows you to match your activity to your mood. For instance, when you're feeling frustrated or angry, you can release those emotions through a highly physical hobby such as metalwork, sculpting or felting. When you're in need of soothing, try a rhythmic, repetitive activity such as knitting, crocheting, cross-stitching or rug-hooking.

• **Share the joy with fellow crafters.** The stress-busting effects of crafting increase synergistically when you combine your hobby with some socializing. To find new friends who share your passion, take a class in your favorite art form or activity...attend a hobbyists' conference...or participate in a crafts fair.

Resource: For an online guide to arts and craft workshops, schools and retreats, visit *www.Art.ShawGuides.com.*

• **Adopt a beginner's mind-set.** Trying to exceed your skill level too fast will only add to your stress, so resist the urge to judge yourself

harshly if a project does not wind up looking like the masterpiece that you originally envisioned. Crafts are not meant to be taken too seriously—that's what the rest of life is for. So don't ruin the fun by being a perfectionist. Instead, focus on the process and not the product...taking pleasure and finding peace in the very act of creating.

Rediscover Your Inner Artist

Cathy A. Malchiodi, PhD, is a research psychologist, art therapist and mental health counselor in Louisville, Kentucky. She is the author of several books, including *The Soul's Palette: Drawing on Art's Transformative Powers for Health and Well-Being*, and a faculty member at Lesley University in Boston.

A seven-year-old asked her mother, "What do you do at work?" The mother replied, "I teach grown-ups to draw." The child stared back, incredulous, and said, "You mean they forgot how?"

It's common to give up on art early in life and lose our natural connection with our inner artist. Innate creativity often is stifled by a developmental shift that occurs around age 10, when we become more conscious of how we are perceived by others...and when others begin to judge us based on our ability to create realistic photolike images, which most people can't do. Girls are particularly approval-oriented, so endeavors that aren't supported—such as expressing ourselves from the heart—fade away.

This is sad. We not only sacrifice the joy of creation, we also miss out on associated health benefits.

Research shows: Artistic activities enhance brain function...alleviate depression...help us cope with pain, illness, loss and trauma...and reduce the stress that can negatively affect physical well-being, including cardiovascular health. So if you have lost touch with your inner artist, today's the day to start the process of rediscovery.

GET INSPIRED

•**Think back to childhood.** Answering the following questions can help you identify the kind of art you want to bring into your life now.

Consider: What artistic activities did you enjoy as a child—drawing, painting, knitting, crafts? What book, movie or natural environment inspired you? Did you prefer to do art alone in your room or backyard, in the kitchen with family members, in a classroom with other artists?

•**Look as if seeing for the first time.** Go to a museum or a place in nature, and look around with fresh eyes. What do you see that you never noticed before? Notice the colors... the textures...the patterns.

•**Observe children as they draw, dance or play-act...**feel their joy, curiosity and lack of inhibition.

•**Come up with a theme that interests you,** such as "What I love," "Life on another planet" or "Nature speaks." Need inspiration? Reread a favorite poem or book.

•**Ignore critics**—inner voices and other people who have told you, "Academics/careers matter more than art" or "Your talents lie elsewhere." Making art isn't about replicating reality, honing technical skills or pleasing others—it's about nourishing your soul through self-expression.

GET READY

•**Gather materials.** Visit an art-supply store and select whatever intrigues you—paper, paints, fabrics, wires, beads, clay, colored tape, etc. Save found objects (shells, twigs), discarded items with interesting shapes (egg cartons, old CDs) or whatever catches your eye—even if you don't know what you might end up doing with them.

•**Choose a special place to store materials, create your art and display your efforts.** To make it a sanctuary, Dr. Malchiodi suggested positioning appealing objects nearby—candles, flowers, prisms, memorabilia, artwork done by others that inspires you.

•**Set aside time in your busy weekly schedule to devote to art...**or if you can, create whenever the spirit moves you.

GET GOING BY EXPERIMENTING WITH...

•**Collage.** Creating a collage is a forgiving first activity because you can keep rearranging things until you are satisfied. It doesn't demand an immediate commitment the way a brushstroke on canvas does.

To make a collage: Tear or cut your materials, rearrange them on the surface of your choice until you find a composition you like, then glue them down...or cut photos, paintings or drawings into strips, then weave them together as you would a mat. You're almost certain to see an interesting result.

•**Clay modeling.** Use potter's clay, Play-Doh or self-hardening clay to express yourself in three dimensions. Close your eyes and press, pull, flatten or mold until you find a shape emerging from the clay...then open your eyes and continue forming the clay until you create a satisfying object. It doesn't look like the statue of David? Who cares?

•**Drawing.** If you feel frustrated when drawings don't turn out as you had hoped, use the following techniques to experience being nonjudgmental of yourself and to make authentic art, not what someone else wants or expects you to do: Draw with your nondominant hand, letting the lines do as they will...or close your eyes and draw without looking at the paper, then see what image emerges...or draw with both hands at once to create mirror images or two completely different pictures.

To "scribble-draw": Tie a string to a stick, dip the string in paint and drag it around on paper until you see an image you like...then color that in.

To "dance-draw": Tape a large piece of craft paper to a wall, put on some music, take a felt-tip marker or chalk in hand and move to the music, transferring your movements to the paper with bold strokes. What you see is a reflection of who you are...and that's art!

C'mon Get Happy

Gretchen Rubin, an attorney and former Supreme Court clerk. Based in New York City, Rubin is founder of The Happiness Project, a blog and newsletter, and author of the best-selling book *The Happiness Project*, for which she personally tested happiness strategies. For more, see Happiness-Project.com.

The philosophers, psychologists and self-help gurus all provide advice on how we can become happier—but what actually works? Journalist Gretchen Rubin decided to find out. She devoted a year to "test-driving" happiness strategies and gathered feedback from visitors to her popular website. She called her research "The Happiness Project."

Different happiness strategies work for different people, but a few strategies stand out...

•**Seek novelty and challenge even if you treasure consistency and comfort.** I did not expect exploring new challenges to make me happier—familiarity and comfort are very important to me—but I was wrong. Trying new things is one of the most effective paths to happiness that I have encountered.

The human brain is stimulated by surprise and discovery. Successfully coping with the unfamiliar can provide a high level of happiness. Repeating what we've done many times before can be comfortable, but comfortable is not the same as happy.

Example: Launching and updating my daily blog have brought me great happiness, though initially I feared that I lacked the necessary technical skills.

Challenge yourself to start something that sounds interesting—even if it's different from anything you've done before or requires skills that you're not sure you have. Take a class...try a new hobby...learn a language...or visit a different town or museum every weekend.

•**Try doing whatever you enjoyed doing at age 10.** The person we are in adulthood has more in common with the person we were at age 10 than we realize. Renowned psychiatrist Carl Jung started playing with building blocks as an adult to recapture some enthusiasm he had felt in his youth. If fishing made us happy when we were 10, odds are it will make us happy today...if playing the drums made us happy then, it probably still will.

Example: I was given a blank book when I was a child and really enjoyed filling it with clippings, notes, cartoons, anything that interested me. So as part of my happiness project, I bought myself a scrapbook and started clipping items from magazines and newspapers to paste into it. I was amazed by how much happiness I still could derive from this.

•**Read memoirs of death and suffering.** Paradoxically, sad memoirs can increase our happiness. These books put our own problems in perspective and remind us how fortunate we are.

Examples: I became much happier with my own life when I read Gene O'Kelly's *Chasing Daylight*, the former CEO's memoir about learning that he had three months to live... Stan Mack's *Janet & Me*, about the death of the author's partner...and Joan Didion's *The Year of Magical Thinking*, about the death of her husband.

It's not that I'm happy that other people have been unhappy. It's just a way of appreciating everything that I do have.

•**De-clutter your home.** Only a few minutes of cleaning up can substantially improve one's mood by giving us the sense that we have accomplished something positive. Cleaning can also create an impression of order that can contribute to serenity. And it helps remove a source of stress—conspicuous clutter is a visual reminder of a responsibility that we have neglected.

Try a brief burst of cleaning the next time you feel overwhelmed or anxious even if you don't think it will work for you. Even people who are not particularly fastidious discover that this boosts their mood.

Examples: For me, cleaning out a drawer...organizing my medicine cabinet...or just making my bed in the morning provides a real boost to my happiness.

•**Be appreciative of people's good traits rather than critical of their bad ones...**be thankful for what they do for you, and stop blaming them for what they don't.

Example: I stopped getting angry at my husband for forgetting to withdraw cash before we went out. Instead, I started taking it upon myself to make sure that we had the necessary cash. I also made a point to be more appreciative of all the things that my husband does do, such as dealing with the car.

• **Enjoy today even if there's still work to do.** Many of us assume it's normal to live with limited happiness until some major milestone is reached—we earn that big promotion, have a family or retire. We tell ourselves, I'll be happy when I achieve my goals.

Example: As a writer, I imagined how happy I would be when the book I was working on was finally published.

Unfortunately, people who pin their happiness on a distant goal usually spend most or all of their lives less happy than they could be. Often they set ever more distant goals as the original targets approach...or they discover that the goal that they thought would bring happiness actually brings added stress. Some never reach their goals at all.

I'm much happier now that I remind myself to be happy about making gradual progress toward my goals, even if the goals themselves remain far in the distance.

Your Gut Can Cause Depression, Arthritis, Diabetes and More

Liz Lipski, PhD, CCN, academic Director of Nutrition and Integrative Health Programs at Maryland University of Integrative Health, is board-certified in clinical nutrition and holistic nutrition. She is the author of several books, including *Digestive Wellness: Strengthen the Immune System and Prevent Disease Through Healthy Digestion*. InnovativeHealing.com.

If you have a stomachache, nausea or some other digestive problem, you know that it stems from your gastrointestinal (GI) tract.

But very few people think of the GI system when they have a health problem such as arthritis, depression, asthma or recurring infections.

Surprising: Tens of millions of Americans are believed to have digestive problems that may not even be recognizable but can cause or complicate many other medical conditions.

Latest development: There's now significant evidence showing just how crucial the digestive system is in maintaining your overall health. How could hidden GI problems be responsible for such a wide range of seemingly unrelated ills?

Here's how: If you can't digest and absorb food properly, your cells can't get the nourishment they need to function properly and you can fall prey to a wide variety of ailments.

Good news: A holistically trained clinician can advise you on natural remedies (available at health-food stores unless otherwise noted) and lifestyle changes that often can correct hidden digestive problems...*

LOW LEVELS OF STOMACH ACID

Stomach acid, which contains powerful, naturally occurring hydrochloric acid (HC1), can decrease due to age, stress and/or food sensitivities.

Adequate stomach acid is a must for killing bacteria, fungi and parasites and for the digestion of protein and minerals. Low levels can weaken immunity and, in turn, lead to problems that can cause or complicate many ailments, including diabetes, gallbladder disease, osteoporosis, rosacea, thyroid problems and autoimmune disorders.

If you suspect that you have low stomach acid: You can be tested by a physician—or simply try the following natural remedies (adding one at a time each week until symptoms improve)...

• **Use apple cider vinegar.** After meals, take one teaspoon in eight teaspoons of water.

• **Try bitters.** This traditional digestive remedy usually contains gentian and other herbs. Bitters, which also are used in mixed drinks, are believed to work by increasing saliva, HC1, pepsin, bile and digestive enzymes. Use as directed on the label in capsule or liquid form.

*Consult your doctor before trying these remedies—especially if you have a chronic medical condition or take any medication.

•**Eat umeboshi plums.** These salted, pickled plums relieve indigestion. Eat them whole as an appetizer or dessert or use umeboshi vinegar to replace vinegar in salad dressings.

•**Take betaine HC1 with pepsin with meals that contain protein.**

Typical dosage: 350 mg. You must be supervised by a health-care professional when using this supplement—it can damage the stomach if used inappropriately.

If you still have symptoms, ask your doctor about adding digestive enzymes such as bromelain and/or papain.

TOO MUCH BACTERIA

When HC1 levels are low, it makes us vulnerable to small intestinal bacterial overgrowth (SIBO). This condition occurs when microbes are introduced into our bodies via our food and cause a low-grade infection or when bacteria from the large intestine migrate into the small intestine, where they don't belong. Left untreated, this bacterial overgrowth can lead to symptoms, such as bloating, gas and changes in bowel movements, characteristic of irritable bowel syndrome (IBS). In fact, some research shows that 78% of people with IBS may actually have SIBO.

SIBO is also a frequent (and usually overlooked) cause of many other health problems, including Crohn's disease, scleroderma (an autoimmune disease of the connective tissue) and fibromyalgia.

SIBO can have a variety of causes, including low stomach acid, overuse of heartburn drugs called proton pump inhibitors (PPIs) and low levels of pancreatic enzymes. Adults over age 65, who often produce less stomach acid, are at greatest risk for SIBO.

Important scientific finding: A study recently conducted by researchers at Washington University School of Medicine found that, for unknown reasons, people with restless legs syndrome are six times more likely to have SIBO than healthy people.

To diagnose: The best test for SIBO is a hydrogen breath test—you drink a sugary fluid and breath samples are then collected. If hydrogen is over-produced, you may have SIBO. The test, often covered by insurance, is offered by gastroenterologists and labs that specialize in digestive tests. For a list of labs that offer at-home tests, visit Siboinfo.com/testing.html.

How to treat: The probiotic VSL-3, available at www.vsl3.com, can be tried. However, antibiotics are usually needed. *Rifaxamin* (Xifaxan) is the antibiotic of choice because it works locally in the small intestine.

LEAKY GUT SYNDROME

The acids and churning action of the stomach blend food into a soupy liquid (chyme) that flows into the small intestine. There, the intestinal lining performs two crucial functions—absorbing nutrients and blocking unwanted substances from entering the bloodstream.

But many factors, such as chronic stress, poor diet, too much alcohol, lack of sleep, and use of antibiotics, prednisone and certain other medications, can inflame and weaken the lining of the small intestine. This allows organisms, such as bacteria, fungi and parasites, and toxic chemicals we encounter in our day-to-day activities, to enter the blood. The problem, called increased intestinal permeability, or leaky gut syndrome, is bad news for the rest of your body.

What happens: The immune system reacts to the organisms and substances as "foreign," triggering inflammation that contributes to or causes a wide range of problems, such as allergies, skin problems, muscle and joint pain, poor memory and concentration, and chronic fatigue syndrome.

To diagnose: A stool test that indicates the presence of parasites, yeast infections or bacterial infection is a sign of leaky gut. So are clinical signs, such as food intolerances and allergies. However, the best test for leaky gut checks for urinary levels of the water-soluble sugars lactulose and mannitol—large amounts indicate a leaky gut.

How to treat: If you and your doctor believe that you have leaky gut, consider taking as many of the following steps as possible...

•**Chew your food slowly and completely to enhance digestion.**

•**Emphasize foods and beverages that can help heal the small intestine,** including foods in the cabbage family, such as kale, vegetable broths, fresh vegetable juices (such as cabbage juice), aloe vera juice and slippery elm tea.

• **Take glutamine.** This amino acid is the main fuel for the small intestine—and a glutamine supplement is one of the best ways to repair a leaky gut. Start with 1 g to 3 g daily, and gradually increase the dosage by a gram or two per week to up to 14 g daily. Becoming constipated is a sign that you're using too much.

• **Try the probiotic L.** plantarum. A supplement of this gut-friendly bacteria, such as Transformation Enzyme's Plantadophilus, can help heal the small intestine.

• **Add quercetin.** This antioxidant helps repair a leaky gut. In my practice, I've found that the products Perque Pain Guard and Perque Repair Guard work better than other quercetin products.

Typical dosage: 1,000 mg daily.

• **Use digestive enzymes with meals to help ensure your food is completely digested.**

Good brands: Enzymedica, Thorne and Now.

GI-RELATED AILMENTS

Health problems linked to poor digestion...

• **Allergies**
• **Arthritis**
• **Asthma**
• **Autoimmune diseases,** such as lupus
• **Depression**
• **Gallbladder disease**
• **Headache**
• **Fatigue**
• **Infections** (recurrent, such as bladder or vaginal)
• **Muscle pain** (chronic)
• **Liver problems**
• **Osteoporosis**
• **Skin conditions,** such as eczema or psoriasis
• **Thyroid problems**

How to Get Unfrazzled

Georgia Witkin, PhD, assistant clinical professor of psychiatry and director of the stress program at Mount Sinai School of Medicine in New York City. She appears on the Fox News Channel and is the author of 10 books, including *The Female Stress Survival Guide.*

As our options have increased over the past few decades, our expectations of ourselves have increased as well. We've added new roles, responsibilities and opportunities—without dropping others.

Result: Our to-do lists are longer than ever. We play catch-up late at night—doing the family's laundry, finishing work assignments, counseling our kids, paying bills for aging parents, e-mailing friends—when what we really need to do is rest.

Being on-call around the clock makes us susceptible to the emotional and the physical costs of stress—from irritability, anxiety and depression to insomnia, headaches, digestive problems and even heart disease.

To keep stress symptoms from becoming chronic, we need to take care of ourselves the same way we take care of others. Of course, when we are pressed for time, it is hard to invest additional time in ourselves. Here's how to feel less overwhelmed—in as little as five seconds.

IF YOU HAVE 5 SECONDS: BREATHE

Focusing on your breathing is the quickest way to interrupt the body's stress reaction. Increased heart rate and blood pressure—two physical stress reactions—are not under voluntary control. But by changing your breathing pattern from fast and shallow to slow and deep, you signal your body to calm down.

Practice belly breathing: Place one hand on your chest and one on your belly button. The hand on your chest should stay still—only the bottom hand should rise and fall. Breathe in...out...and pause. This sequence should take about five seconds. For greater benefit, repeat 10 times.

Option: Close your eyes and imagine your breath as a mist of your favorite color. This engages the visual part of your brain, switching attention away from the worrying words inside your head.

IF YOU HAVE 5 MINUTES: MOVE

Physical activity burns off adrenaline that floods your body when you're overwhelmed.

Best: Dancing, which restores a stress-relieving sense of control—you hear the rhythm of the music and know the next beat will follow a predictable pattern.

Keep a portable music player and earphones handy, and move to your favorite music for five minutes.

Important: The music should be fast—faster than the average heartbeat of 72 beats a minute. Although slow music can be calming when you're already relaxed, it's likely to frustrate you when you're frantic.

IF YOU HAVE 5 HOURS: PLAY

Regularly set aside a few hours to do whatever helps you feel renewed.

- **Browse in a bookstore**
- **Get a massage or facial**
- **Go for a long walk in the woods**
- **Take an art class**

Once a week is ideal, but even once a month helps. Don't feel guilty—these breaks promote physical and emotional health and give you more energy to tackle whatever tasks await you afterward.

Trap to avoid: Using scheduled playtime to catch up with chores, errands or correspondence. If you can't resist the temptation to work instead of play, take your break outside the house, away from reminders of all that needs to be done. You can include family as long as the activity is genuinely fun for you and easy to arrange. If you can't spare five hours, take an hour or two this week and promise yourself extra playtime next week.

IF YOU HAVE 5 DAYS: ESCAPE

Family outings and extended trips can be fun but often add to stress—because wives and mothers usually wind up planning, packing and keeping track of everyone's needs during the trip.

Solution: Take a mini-vacation with a girlfriend or by yourself. At least five days is ideal because it takes most people a few days to wind down and let go of work and home concerns.

What if you can only manage a weekend or long weekend? For several days beforehand, take a few minutes each morning and evening to visualize yourself at your destination—stretched out on the beach, strolling through a museum or enjoying a fabulous meal.

IN 5 WEEKS: FORM NEW HABITS

For a long-term approach to strengthening your self-care skills, develop a new stress-reducing behavior each week.

Week 1: **Practice saying no.** Turn down all non-emergency requests for help. Don't apologize. Say graciously but matter-of-factly, "Thanks for asking, but I'm overextended and have to say no." At the end of the week, when and if you start to say yes again, you'll be more discriminating about the responsibilities you agree to take on.

Week 2: **Prune your to-do list.** Whenever you add a task to your list, cross off another either by delegating it or letting it go. Each evening, erase one nonessential uncompleted task. When an unexpected hassle arises, such as the car breaking down, cross off two or three items—it doesn't matter if your closets stay cluttered or your dinner-party desserts aren't homemade.

Week 3: **Mother yourself.** Whatever loving care you would provide for a child, do for yourself. Feed yourself well...take a nap...enjoy some physical activity...get eight hours of sleep every night...pay yourself a compliment when you need one.

Week 4: **Act "as if."** It's not necessary to feel comfortable with a change before you can shift behavior—when you change behavior first, feelings follow. The more you treat yourself as if you're entitled to play and take breaks and say no, the more genuinely entitled you'll feel. Act as though other people are delighted to treat you the way you want to be treated. Soon you'll feel comfortable asking for what you need and will respond to others' helpfulness with appreciation rather than guilt.

Week 5: **Change your internal dialog.** Every time you catch yourself thinking "I should..." substitute, "It would be nice if I could..." or

109

"How terrific that my sister is able to..." Then follow with, "It's okay for me not to..." With practice, you'll start to believe it—and you'll stop feeling frazzled.

6 Foods Proven to Make You Happy: One Tops Antidepressants

Tonia Reinhard, MS, RD, a registered dietitian and professor at Wayne State University in Detroit. She is the program director for the Coordinated Program in Dietetics, course director of clinical nutrition at Wayne State University School of Medicine and past president of the Michigan Academy of Nutrition and Dietetics. She is author of *Superfoods: The Healthiest Foods on the Planet* and *SuperJuicing: More Than 100 Nutritious Vegetable & Fruit Recipes*.

You can eat your way to a better mood! Certain foods and beverages have been proven to provide the raw materials that you need to feel sharper, more relaxed and just plain happier. *Best choices...*

HAPPY FOOD #1:
CHOCOLATE

Chocolate can make you feel good—to such an extent that 52% of women would choose chocolate over sex, according to one survey.

Chocolate contains chemical compounds known as polyphenols, which interact with neurotransmitters in the brain and reduce anxiety. An Australian study found that men and women who consumed the most chocolate polyphenols (in the form of a beverage) felt calmer and more content than those who consumed a placebo drink.

Chocolate also boosts serotonin, the same neurotransmitter affected by antidepressant medications. It triggers the release of dopamine and stimulates the "pleasure" parts of the brain.

Then there's the sensual side of chocolate—the intensity of the flavor and the melting sensation as it dissolves in your mouth. The satisfaction that people get from chocolate could be as helpful for happiness as its chemical composition.

Recommended amount: Aim for one ounce of dark chocolate a day. Most studies used dark chocolate with 70% cacao or more.

HAPPY FOOD #2:
FISH

Fish has been called "brain food" because our brains have a high concentration of omega-3 fatty acids—and so does fish. These fatty acids have been linked to memory and other cognitive functions. In countries where people eat a lot of fish, depression occurs less often than in countries (such as the US) where people eat less.

The omega-3s in fish accumulate in the brain and increase "membrane fluidity," the ability of brain-cell membranes to absorb nutrients and transmit chemical signals.

A study out of Harvard Medical School published in *Archives of General Psychiatry* looked at patients diagnosed with depression who hadn't responded well to antidepressants. Those who were given 1,000 mg of EPA (a type of omega-3 fatty acid) daily for three months had significant improvements, including less anxiety and better sleep.

Recommended amount: Try to have at least two or three fish meals a week. Cold-water fish—such as sardines, mackerel and salmon—have the highest levels of omega-3s. Or choose a supplement with 1,000 mg of EPA and DHA (another omega-3 fatty acid) in total.

HAPPY FOOD #3:
DARK GREEN VEGGIES

Dark green vegetables such as spinach, asparagus, broccoli and Brussels sprouts are loaded with folate, a B-complex vitamin that plays a key role in regulating mood. A Harvard study found that up to 38% of adults with depression had low or borderline levels of folate. Boosting the folate levels of depressed patients improved their mood.

Dark green vegetables are particularly good, but all vegetables and fruits boost mood. Researchers asked 281 people to note their moods on different days. On the days when the participants consumed the most vegetables and fruits, they reported feeling happier and more energetic. Folate certainly plays a role, but self-satisfaction may have something to do with it as well. People feel good when they eat right and take care of themselves.

Recommended amount: The minimum you should have is five servings of vegetables and fruits a day.

Bonus: Middle-aged men who had 10 servings a day showed reduced blood pressure.

HAPPY FOOD #4:
BEANS (INCLUDING SOYBEANS)

Beans are rich in tryptophan, an essential amino acid that is used by the body to produce serotonin, the neurotransmitter that affects feelings of calmness and relaxation.

Beans also are loaded with folate. Folate, as mentioned in the veggies section, plays a key role in regulating mood.

In addition, beans contain manganese, a trace element that helps prevent mood swings due to low blood sugar.

Recommended amount: For people not used to eating beans, start with one-quarter cup five days a week. Build up to one-half cup daily. This progression will help prevent gastrointestinal symptoms such as flatulence.

HAPPY FOOD #5:
NUTS

Nuts are high in magnesium, a trace mineral involved in more than 300 processes in the body. People who don't get enough magnesium feel irritable, fatigued and susceptible to stress.

The elderly are more likely than young adults to be low in magnesium—because they don't eat enough magnesium-rich foods and/or because they tend to excrete more magnesium in their urine.

Also, many health problems can accelerate the depletion of magnesium from the body.

Examples: Gastrointestinal disorders (or bariatric surgery), kidney disease and sometimes diabetes.

Recommended amount: Aim for one ounce of nuts a day. Good choices include almonds, walnuts, cashews, hazelnuts and peanuts (the latter is technically a legume). If you don't like nuts, other high-magnesium foods include spinach, pumpkin seeds, fish, beans, whole grains and dairy.

HAPPY FOOD #6:
COFFEE

The caffeine in coffee, tea and other caffeinated beverages is a very beneficial compound. One study found that people with mild cognitive impairment were less likely to develop full-fledged Alzheimer's disease when they had the caffeine equivalent of about three cups of coffee a day.

Caffeine can temporarily improve your memory and performance on tests. It enhances coordination and other parameters of physical performance. When you feel energized, you feel happier. Also, people who feel good from caffeine may be more likely to engage in other happiness-promoting behaviors, such as seeing friends and exercising.

Recommended amount: The challenge is finding the "sweet spot"—just enough caffeine to boost mood but not so much that you get the shakes or start feeling anxious. For those who aren't overly sensitive to caffeine, one to three daily cups of coffee or tea are about right.

WHAT NOT TO EAT

Some people turn to food or drink for comfort when they're feeling down. *Here's what not to eat or drink when you've got the blues…*

• **Alcohol.** Alcohol is a depressant of the central nervous system. When you initially consume alcohol, it produces a euphoric effect and you become more animated and less inhibited. But as you continue drinking and more alcohol crosses the blood-brain barrier, the depressant effect predominates.

• **Baked goods.** When you eat high-sugar, high-fat carbs such as cookies, pastries and donuts, you tend to want more of them. The food gives you a temporary "good feeling," but the excess food intake that typically results causes drowsiness and often self-loathing.

If You Don't Want to Take an Antidepressant...

Jamison Starbuck, ND, is a naturopathic physician in family practice and a guest lecturer at the University of Montana, both in Missoula. She is past president of the American Association of Naturopathic Physicians and a contributing editor to *The Alternative Advisor: The Complete Guide to Natural Therapies and Alternative Treatments.*

"I don't want to take these pills anymore!" Janet said, holding up a plastic prescription bottle and shaking it vigorously. "I don't like how they make me feel!" The drug was *fluoxetine* (Prozac), and the scenario is one with which I have become very familiar.

Like Janet, today more than 10% of Americans take an antidepressant. Even though antidepressants can sometimes be life-saving—for example, if a person feels suicidal—these drugs are prescribed, in my opinion, to far too many people. Less than 32% of patients who take antidepressants see mental health professionals. Family physicians often prescribe antidepressants for mild depression, anxiety and premenstrual syndrome. In addition, the drugs may be prescribed inappropriately when a physical problem, such as a hormone imbalance, is causing the depressive symptoms.

Many of my patients who have taken an antidepressant say that the drug makes them feel flat. Life may be less fraught with fear or anger for these people, but it often becomes—to them—monotonous and even dull. Common side effects also may include a lack of interest in sex, an inability to focus and an increased tendency to procrastinate. Based on my patients' experiences, in some cases, these drugs may cause personality changes that adversely influence relationships, job choices and self-esteem.

In my practice, I have helped hundreds of people transition off antidepressants and move forward in medication-free, depression-free lives.

Very important: If you would like to stop taking an antidepressant, do so only with the help of a physician—withdrawal symptoms may occur.

Advice I've given to my patients who want to give up antidepressants...

•**Find a safe way to express your inner emotional state.** When you reduce your antidepressant medication, your emotions will be more strongly felt. In my opinion, these emotions are best examined in therapy with a mental health professional. However, I've seen patients work with their emotions in lots of ways—for example, through dance, journaling, music, weekly meetings with a pastor or close personal friend.

•**Try tryptophan.** This amino acid is used by the body to make serotonin, a calming brain chemical. Though not as strong as synthetic antidepressants, tryptophan works well for mild-to-moderate anxiety and depression. If a person is transitioning off of an antidepressant, I often initially prescribe 500 mg of L-tryptophan two times a day, 30 minutes away from food, on alternating days with the prescription medication.

•**Take pantothenic acid (vitamin B-5).** This vitamin enhances function of the adrenal glands, which help us manage stress.

Typical dose: 250 mg twice daily with food.

•**Consider using Gotu kola,** an herb that improves circulation to the brain and calms the nervous system. If a person is going off of an antidepressant, I typically recommend 30 drops of tincture in two ounces of water, 30 minutes before or after meals, four times a day for four to six weeks.

The Artist's Way to Heart Health

Harlan M. Krumholz, MD, professor of medicine and epidemiology and public health (cardiology), section of cardiovascular medicine, Yale University School of Medicine, New Haven, Connecticut.

Remember when, as a child, you happily drew and painted pictures and made clay animals? Remember the pure delight in picking out a tune on the piano, dancing without caring what others thought and writing stories and poems? Few of us continue those creative pursuits into adulthood…but perhaps we should. Medical experts now are studying how artistic expression can improve heart health—in fact, it can be prescribed right along with exercise, healthy diet and medicines for patients with cardiovascular disease or at risk for it. Can you picture it—instead of a prescription for statins or a hypertension drug, your doctor sends you home with instructions to make a collage?

There's a definite connection between creative expression and healing. Studies have demonstrated that acute or chronic stress can increase the risk for cardiovascular disease. We know, for example, that the acute emotional distress of broken heart syndrome can damage the heart, stress from events like earthquakes can cause a spike in the number of heart attacks and, similarly, the trauma of serious illness can shock your system, as it makes you aware of your vulnerability and mortality.

ART & YOUR HEART: HAPPY TOGETHER

Art can be a way to reduce such stress. If stress is bad for you, then creative pursuits are the opposite—creative pursuits allow people to find their "flow state," a mental state in which they are so fully involved in an activity that they become unaware of passing time. Stress and flow are mutually exclusive—spending time unstressed, with the benefits of lower blood pressure, lower heart rate and deeper respiration improves immune function, reduces anxiety and worry and can result in reduced risk for heart disease.

The mind-body connection is fascinating, and heart disease, in particular, has a special connection with the mind. We're too often leaping to the next drug. It's valuable to explore how lifestyle strategies such as engaging in creative arts may favorably influence risk.

WHAT SCIENTISTS KNOW

A considerable body of evidence supports these ideas. *We already know…*

• **Art helps you to process feelings about experiences that are too difficult to put into words,** and it also can be a refuge from the intense emotion associated with illness. In a study of women with cancer, researchers found that working with textiles and making cards, collages, pottery, watercolors or acrylics helped relieve participants of their preoccupation with illness while also enhancing their self-worth. Their artistic endeavors provided opportunities for achievement…gave them a social identity that was not defined by their cancer…and allowed them to express feelings that might otherwise be too upsetting to face.

• **Dance and creative movement bring mind/body benefits.** Music has the power to change how you feel, as we all have experienced…and avid athletes know that endorphins (brain chemicals created during exercise) improve mood. Combining these two can be a way to express your emotions while also realizing the health benefits of music and exercise.

• **Writing about traumatic experiences produces significant improvements in mood and health.** Dozens of studies have shown that "emotional writing" (also called expressive writing) can reduce frequency of doctor visits, improve immune function, reduce levels of stress hormones and blood pressure, and lift a depressed mood. You can try journaling, poetry or just jotting down your thoughts, and you don't need to worry about editing yourself—it's the process of being creative and expressive that's so valuable.

EXPRESS YOURSELF!

You can start applying this premise to your life now. There's no limit to the ways you can engage in art in your life. Find a pursuit that fits your interests, and don't worry about how others judge your performance. Everyone has an inner life, ideas, and a capacity to be artistic in some way. Just as with the children who draw, paint and sing simply because they like doing it, this is all about the process, not the product. Your art doesn't have to be "good" to be good for you. Free the artist within.. and see what a difference it can make!

Three Easy Steps to Access Your Creativity

Julia Cameron, author of the popular book *The Artist's Way* and more recently, *The Writing Diet*. In addition to a successful career as playwright, screenwriter, author and more, Cameron has for many years taught creativity workshops.

Do you envy people who are naturally creative—artists, musicians, poets and the like? Don't make the mistake of overlooking computer programmers, schoolteachers, doctors or receptionists. In our society we often assume creativity belongs only to a select few, those who dwell in the so-called world of "the arts." But creativity exists in all of us. It is simply having the ability to come up with new and original ideas—the very talent needed to run businesses, raise families and turn everyday life into a richer, more interesting and enjoyable experience. For people contemplating a transition from one way of living to another…retiring, perhaps, or changing professions or even getting a divorce, it is essential to create your new life.

When faced with life change, few people realize creativity is critical to their success—nor how to harness and use it to their benefit. Julia Cameron, author of the popular book *The Artist's Way* and more recently, *The Writing Diet*, has had a successful career as playwright, screenwriter, author and more. For many years she taught creativity workshops that attract a wide range of people. She has developed a method that has helped her students tap into their creativity. It mostly consists of three easy-to-do activities—but, she emphasizes, they require diligence and commitment in order to make a difference in your life.

STEP ONE: THE MORNING PAGES

Most people's early morning involves equal parts coffee and the news. Step one revises old habits by introducing a new early morning ritual—the morning pages. Each day upon arising, sit down and write three pages in a notebook—not two or four but three. Write about whatever you like—your dreams from the night before, the moods you've been in of late, your anger or enchantment with someone

you know…you can fantasize or whine—or both…you can plan or free associate—or both. These pages are yours. Cameron explains that eventually your morning pages will guide you to creative venues you would otherwise be blind to. "They move people into confidence and adventure," she says, adding that nothing is too grand or too petty to be included in the pages. They are for your eyes only, "to vent, to plan, to dream, to mourn, to complain, to explore. They acquaint people with how they really feel," she says…and they become what she describes as the "greased slide to all other forms of creativity."

For the morning pages you will need a fresh notebook (and they fill up fast) and a comfortable place to sit quietly. Privacy is extremely important when doing the pages because in them you meet yourself, uninterrupted or interpreted by others. It may take days or weeks to get the hang of filling three pages…in the meantime feel free to repeat yourself or write nonsense.

Morning pages are meant to be a lifelong habit. Writing early in the day, Cameron claims, somehow settles your mind and helps you develop priorities, instead of having vague thoughts buzz around in your head all day that go nowhere. She believes they bring clarity so it doesn't take long to see your "authentic self" begin to emerge in the pages, along with its hopes and dreams through repeated themes—take good care of them because they reflect your creativity at work. "Ideas come to people in their pages that at first seem impossible," says Cameron, "but then the pages start to move their ideas into the arena of possible."

STEP TWO: ARTIST'S DATES

In step two, Cameron has created something she calls "Artist's Dates." These are meant to give you an adventure every week. It can be as mundane as going to a carpet shop to admire the oriental rugs or a greenhouse to enjoy the flora. You might visit a spice store to experience the colors and smells, or a fabric store to gaze at and touch the plethora of designs and textures. You could walk through an unfamiliar church, take a hike or go to a new restaurant with exotic foods. Where you go and what you see doesn't matter. These visits are intended to stimulate your senses in new and unusual ways (at least new and unusual for you) and they allow your playful side to have fun—in fact, says Cameron, these outings are meant to teach people how to play.

Surprisingly, people fear they can't come up with ideas for artist date outings. The problem is, Cameron says, they're confusing them with high art. Not so, she says, they are silly, frivolous and meant to let the imagination play. To generate ideas about outings that appeal to you, she suggests taking a blank page and quickly writing down 10 things you could do. Following through each week with your dates will enrich your inner life. Think of yourself as an ecosystem, working to keep your creative pond well stocked. Your artist's dates will do just that. They can be brief or last all day—but are best done solo so you can focus on the experience.

STEP THREE: REGULAR WALKS

Take regular walks alone. Although Cameron has made a habit of frequent walking, it took her many years to recognize how productive walks are for creativity.

The reason: Walking by yourself provides the peacefulness you need to integrate your insights. Morning pages send messages about what you do and do not like…your artist's dates allow you to take in things that are of interest to you…and walking is the ideal time to merge what you have learned. Cameron has found that it takes about 20 minutes of walking to move into a more imaginative state, and so she advises doing so for a minimum of 20 minutes, at least once a week. However, once you are in that imaginative state, you may want to extend your walk to an hour or so. And you may choose to walk much more often…for your creativity and your health.

While you walk, it's important to turn off your cell phone. "The idea isn't to tune out… it's to tune in," says Cameron. Your pages and dates will stimulate your creative voice—the quiet walks provide a chance to hear everything it has to say.

3 Easy Art Projects Anyone Can Do

Amy Cohen, an artist and art teacher based in New York City. She has more than 30 years of experience as a private art instructor and portfolio consultant for aspiring art school students. AmyArtCohen.com

Some people avoid artistic endeavors because they don't consider themselves skilled at drawing or painting. But even people who lack technical artistic skills can create works of art.

Bonus: Engaging in the artistic process can relieve stress, spur creative thinking and boost self-esteem.

Three fun art projects…

COLLAGE

Collages are artistic compositions created by combining things such as photographs, scraps of paper featuring distinctive graphics or drawings and small swatches of fabric.

First, collect materials that appeal to you. You can do this by buying old books containing evocative photos or drawings in thrift stores or at library book sales…saving small pieces of attractive or interesting wrapping paper or cloth…and/or saving product packaging that includes distinctive graphics. I don't recommend saving images from modern magazines—they're not particularly intriguing.

Next, cut out elements from the materials you have collected, and glue them to a paper backing in combinations or patterns that you find compelling. Use heavy-weight drawing paper—look for "Bristol" paper—and an acid-free glue stick. These are available in art-supply stores, craft stores and even some office-supply stores. Don't use standard Elmer's glue or a child's glue stick—these could discolor or otherwise damage the materials.

Some collage artists create collages with specific themes, perhaps forming a nature scene by combining an image of a tree, a photo of a fish and a piece of blue cloth to represent a lake. Other collage artists pull together materials that have no particular thematic connection. If you are not sure how to start, just pick an image that you find compelling, cut it out, glue it to a page, then find another image that you think looks good when paired with it and repeat the process. Keep doing this, and see where it leads.

Helpful: The book *Cut & Paste: 21st-Century Collage* by Richard Brereton and Caroline Roberts is full of interesting collage ideas. Or search the Web for the word "collage" together with the names of artists Hannah Höch and/or Max Ernst to find collage examples to use as inspiration.

SODA CAN ART

Art projects made with soda or beer cans often appeal to people who don't consider themselves artistic, because they involve skills such as hammering and metal cutting that are very different from the classical academic art skills of drawing and painting. Start by looking through your empty soda or beer cans before taking them to be recycled. Save any that have colors and graphics that you find appealing. Use tin snips or a strong pair of scissors to cut off the tops and bottoms of these cans, then cut open the cylinders. Unroll the cylinders, and press them flat under something heavy, such as a stack of books.

Warning: Wear sturdy work gloves while cutting aluminum to avoid getting cut by the metal's sharp edges.

Next, use small nails to affix a piece of aluminum flashing onto a rectangular piece of wood. Rolls of silver aluminum flashing can be purchased in home stores, often for less than $1 per square foot. Cut this aluminum so that it completely covers one side of the wood.

Once your cans have been pressed flat, cut shapes or patterns out of them, then use small nails to attach these pieces of colored aluminum onto the aluminum flashing to create distinctive metallic art. You can use the colored aluminum to create patterns or even to construct pictures.

Search on the web for "soda can art" to view examples of projects.

DUCT TAPE ART

Duct tape might seem utilitarian and prosaic, but this well-known adhesive product now is available in a wide range of colors and patterns in art-supply stores and crafts stores.

If you purchase a selection of duct tape in different colors, you can combine them to create eye-catching artwork and crafts without ever touching a paintbrush or pen. My students, ages six to 90, love it!

Duck brand duct tape lists some of these arts and crafts projects on the company's website. (On *www.DuckBrand.com*, click on Crafts & Decor).

You can create duct tape pictures with strips of duct tape on a piece of plywood or heavy cardboard. Or you can layer different colors. Then use a sharp craft knife to cut out sections of the top layer(s) and peel them away to expose the colors below.

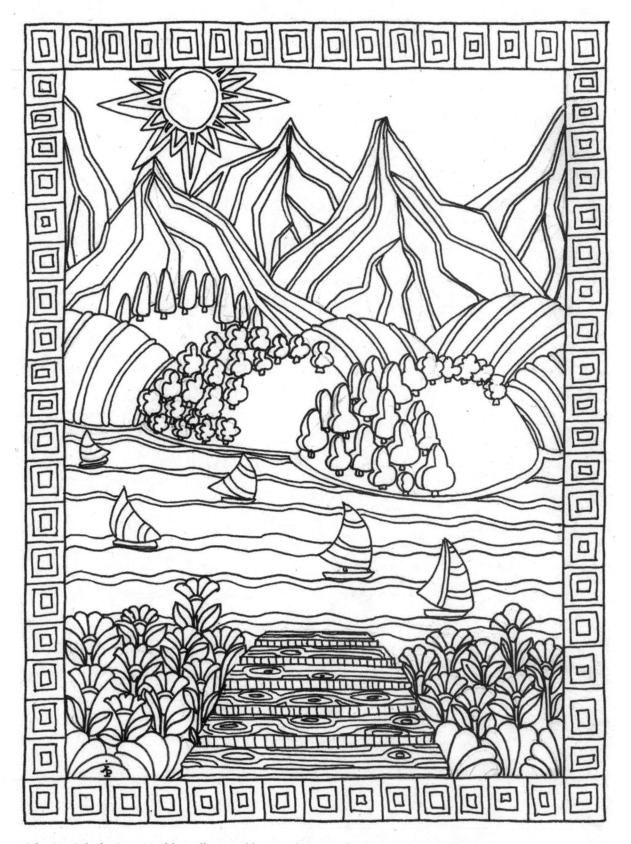

Color Me Calm by Lacy Mucklow, illustrated by Angela Porter (2015, Race Point Publishing).

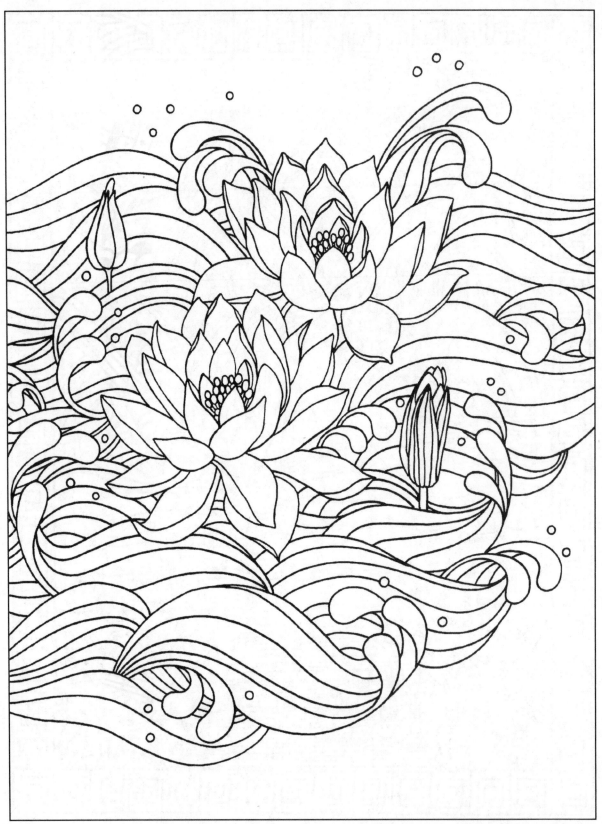

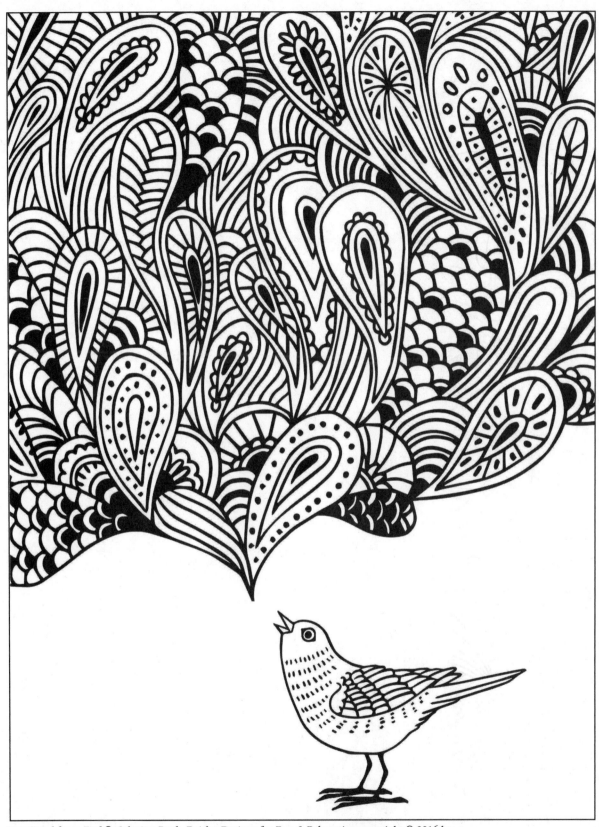

119

8

Throw Away Your Diabetes Medications!

How America's Top Diabetes Doctor Avoids Diabetes

You might think that a diabetes researcher would never develop the disease that he's dedicated his life to studying. But I can't count on it.

My family's story: My father was diagnosed with diabetes at age 72 and was promptly placed on three medications to control his insulin levels.

What he did next made all the difference: Even though he began taking diabetes medication, he simultaneously went into action—walking an hour a day and going on the diet described below. A year and a half later, he no longer needed the prescriptions. He still had diabetes, but diet and exercise kept it under control.

As a diabetes researcher and physician whose own diabetes risk is increased by his family his-

tory, I've got a lot at stake in finding the absolute best ways to avoid and fight this disease.

Here are the steps I take to prevent diabetes—all of which can benefit you whether you want to avoid this disease or have already been diagnosed with it and are trying to control or even reverse it…

STEP 1: **Follow a rural Asian diet (RAD).** This diet includes the most healthful foods of a traditional Asian diet—it consists of 70% complex carbohydrates…15% fat…15% protein…and 15 g of fiber for every 1,000 calories. Don't worry too much about all these numbers—the diet is actually pretty simple to follow once you get the hang of it.

You might be surprised by "70% complex carbohydrates," since most doctors recommend lower daily intakes of carbohydrates. The difference is, I'm recommending high amounts

---

George L. King, MD, chief scientific officer at the Boston-based Joslin Diabetes Center, one of the country's leading diabetes clinical care and research centers. He is also a professor of medicine at Harvard Medical School and the author, with Royce Flippin, of *The Diabetes Reset*.

of complex, unrefined (not processed) carbo-hydrates. This type of carb is highly desirable because it's found in foods—such as whole grains, legumes, vegetables and fruits—that are chock-full of fiber. If your goal is to reduce diabetes risk, fiber is the holy grail.

Why I do it: The RAD diet has been proven in research to promote weight loss…improve insulin sensitivity (a key factor in the develop-ment and treatment of diabetes) and glucose control…and decrease total cholesterol and LDL "bad" cholesterol levels.

To keep it simple, I advise patients to follow a 2-1-1 formula when creating meals—two por-tions of nonstarchy veggies (such as spinach, carrots or asparagus)…one portion of whole grains (such as brown rice or quinoa), legumes (such as lentils or chickpeas) or starchy veggies (such as sweet potatoes or winter squash)… and one portion of protein (such as salmon, lean beef, tofu or eggs). Have a piece of fruit (such as an apple or a pear) on the side. Por-tion size is also important. Portions fill a nine-inch-diameter plate, which is smaller than a typical 12-inch American dinner plate.

Helpful: I take my time when eating—I chew each bite at least 10 times before swal-lowing. Eating too quickly can cause glucose levels to peak higher than usual after a meal.

STEP 2: **Fill up on dark green vegetables.** I include dark, leafy greens in my diet every day. These leafy greens are one of the two portions of nonstarchy veggies in the 2-1-1 formula.

Why I do it: Dark green vegetables contain antioxidants and compounds that help your body fight insulin resistance (a main driver of diabetes).

My secret "power veggie": A Chinese veg-etable called bitter melon. It is a good source of fiber and has been shown to lower blood sugar. True to its name, bitter melon tastes a little bitter but is delicious when used in soups and stir-fries. It is available at Asian groceries. Eat bitter melon as one of the two portions of nonstarchy veggies in the 2-1-1 formula.

STEP 3: **Adopt an every-other-day work-out routine.** I try to not be sedentary and to walk as much as I can (by using a pedometer, I can tell whether I've reached my daily goal of 10,000 steps).

While this daily practice helps, it's not enough to significantly affect my diabetes risk. For that, I have an every-other-day workout routine that consists of 30 minutes of jogging on the tread-mill (fast enough so that I'm breathing hard but can still carry on a conversation)…followed by 30 minutes of strength training (using handheld weights, resistance bands or weight machines).

Why I do it: Working out temporarily re-duces your insulin resistance and activates enzymes and proteins that help your muscles use glucose instead of allowing the body to accumulate fat—a beneficial effect that lasts for 48 hours (the reason for my every-other-day routine). Strength training is crucial—your muscles are what really kick your body's glu-cose-burning into high gear. A weekly game of tennis helps shake up my routine.

STEP 4: **Keep the temperature chilly.** At the courts where I play tennis, the tempera-ture is naturally cool, but I wear a very thin T-shirt that leaves my neck exposed. This helps activate the "brown fat" in my body. Most peo-ple have this special type of body fat—mainly around the neck, collarbone and shoulders.

Why I do it: Brown fat burns calories at high rates when triggered by the cold. To help burn brown fat, exercise in temperatures of 64°F or lower…set your home's thermostat in the mid-60s…and dress as lightly as possible in cool weather. Walking for 50 or 60 minutes a day in cool weather also helps.

STEP 5: **Get the "sleep cure."** I make a point to sleep at least six hours a night during the week and seven hours nightly on weekends.

Why I do it: Lack of sleep has been prov-en to dramatically harm the body's ability to properly metabolize glucose—a problem that sets the stage for diabetes. Research shows that seven to eight hours a night are ideal. How-ever, because of my work schedule, I'm not al-ways able to get that much sleep on weekdays. That's why I sleep a bit longer on weekends.

Research now shows that the body has some capacity to "catch up" on lost sleep and reverse some—but not all-—of the damage that occurs to one's insulin sensitivity when you're sleep deprived.

Fight Diabetes Naturally: Three Proven Nondrug Remedies

Bill Gottlieb, CHC, a health coach certified by the American Association of Drugless Practitioners. He is author of 13 health books that have sold more than two million copies and former editor in chief of Rodale Books and *Prevention Magazine Health Books*. BillGottliebHealth.com

Scientific research and the experience of doctors and other health professionals show that supplements and superfoods can be even more effective than drugs when it comes to preventing and treating diabetes. I reviewed thousands of scientific studies and talked to more than 60 health professionals about these glucose-controlling natural remedies. One is magnesium. Studies show that magnesium significantly reduces the risk for diabetes. (*Note*: High doses of magnesium can cause diarrhea.)

Here are three more standout natural remedies…

Caution: If you are taking insulin or other medications to control diabetes, talk to your doctor before taking any supplement or changing your diet.

GYMNEMA

Gymnema has been the standard antidiabetes recommendation for the past 2,000 years from practitioners of Ayurveda, the ancient system of natural healing from India. Derived from a vinelike plant found in the tropical forests of southern and central India, the herb also is called gurmar, or "sugar destroyer"—if you chew on the leaf of the plant, you temporarily will lose your ability to taste sweets.

Modern science has figured out the molecular interactions underlying this strange phenomenon. The gymnemic acids in the herb have a structure similar to glucose molecules, filling up glucose receptor sites on the taste buds. They also fill up sugar receptors in the intestine, blocking the absorption of glucose. And gymnemic acids stimulate (and even may regenerate) the cells of the pancreas that man-ufacture insulin, the hormone that ushers glucose out of the bloodstream and into cells.

Standout research: Studies published in Journal of Ethnopharmacology showed that three months of using a unique gymnema extract, formulated over several decades by two Indian scientists, reduced fasting blood glucose (a blood sample is taken after an overnight fast) by 23% in people with type 2 diabetes (defined as fasting blood sugar levels of 126 mg/dL or higher). People with prediabetes (defined as those with blood sugar levels of 100 mg/dL to 125 mg/dL) had a 30% reduction.

Important: The newest (and more powerful) version of this extract is called ProBeta, which is available at PharmaTerra.com. A naturopathic physician who uses ProBeta with his patients told me that the supplement can lower fasting glucose in the 200s down to the 120s or 130s after five to six months of use.

Typical daily dose: ProBeta—two capsules, two to three times a day. Other types of gymnema—400 milligrams (mg), three times a day.

APPLE CIDER VINEGAR

Numerous studies have proved that apple cider vinegar works to control type 2 diabetes. Several of the studies were conducted by Carol Johnston, PhD, RD, a professor of nutrition at Arizona State University.

Standout scientific research: Dr. Johnston's studies showed that an intake of apple cider vinegar with a meal lowered insulin resistance (the inability of cells to use insulin) by an average of 64% in people with prediabetes and type 2 diabetes…improved insulin sensitivity (the ability of cells to use insulin) by up to 34%…and lowered postmeal spikes in blood sugar by an average of 20%. Research conducted in Greece, Sweden, Japan and the Middle East has confirmed many of Dr. Johnston's findings.

How it works: The acetic acid in vinegar—the compound that gives vinegar its tart flavor and pungent odor—blunts the activity of disaccharidase enzymes that help break down the type of carbohydrates found in starchy foods such as potatoes, rice, bread and pasta. As a result, those foods are digested and absorbed more slowly, lowering blood glucose and insulin levels.

Suggested daily intake: Two tablespoons right before or early in the meal. (More is not more effective.)

If you're using vinegar in a salad dressing, the ideal ratio for blood sugar control is two tablespoons of vinegar to one tablespoon of oil. Eat the salad early in the meal so that it disrupts the carb-digesting enzymes before they get a chance to work. Or dip premeal whole-grain bread in a vinaigrette dressing.

SOY FOODS

A new 10-year study published in *Journal of the American Society of Nephrology* found that the mortality rate for people with diabetes and kidney disease was more than 31%. Statistically, that makes kidney disease the number-one risk factor for death in people with diabetes.

Fortunately, researchers have found that there is a simple way to counter kidney disease in diabetes—eat more soy foods.

Standout scientific research: Dozens of scientific studies show that soy is a nutritional ally for diabetes patients with kidney disease. But the best and most recent of these studies, published in Diabetes Care, shows that eating lots of soy can help reverse signs of kidney disease, reduce risk factors for heart disease—and reduce blood sugar, too.

The study involved 41 diabetes patients with kidney disease, divided into two groups. One group ate a diet with protein from 70% animal and 30% vegetable sources. The other group ate a diet with protein from 35% animal sources, 35% textured soy protein and 30% vegetable proteins. After four years, those eating the soy-rich diet had lower levels of several biomarkers for kidney disease. (In another, smaller experiment, the same researchers found that soy improved biomarkers for kidney disease in just seven weeks.) In fact, the health of the participants' kidneys actually improved, a finding that surprised the researchers, since diabetic nephropathy (diabetes-caused kidney disease) is considered to be a progressive, irreversible disease.

Those eating soy also had lower fasting blood sugar, lower LDL cholesterol, lower total cholesterol, lower triglycerides and lower C-reactive protein, a biomarker for chronic inflammation.

How it works: Substituting soy for animal protein may ease stress on the delicate filters of the kidneys. Soy itself also stops the overproduction of cells in the kidney that clog the filters...boosts the production of nitric oxide, which improves blood flow in the kidneys... and normalizes the movement of minerals within the kidneys, thus improving filtration.

Suggested daily intake: The diabetes patients in the study ate 16 grams of soy protein daily.

Examples: Four ounces of tofu provide 13 grams of soy protein...one soy burger, 13 grams...one-quarter cup of soy nuts, 11 grams...one-half cup of shelled edamame (edible soybeans in the pod), 11 grams...one cup of soy milk, 6 grams.

WHAT'S WRONG WITH DIABETES DRUGS?

Doctors typically try to control high blood sugar with a glucose-lowering medication such as *metformin* (Glucophage), a drug most experts consider safe. But other diabetes drugs may not be safe.

Example #1: Recent studies show that *sitagliptin* (Januvia) and *exenatide* (Byetta) double the risk for hospitalization for pancreatitis (inflamed pancreas) and triple the risk for pancreatic cancer.

Example #2: *Pioglitazone* (Actos) can triple the risk for eye problems and vision loss, double the risk for bone fractures in women and double the risk for bladder cancer.

Say Good-Bye to Your Diabetes Medication

Mark A. Stengler, NMD, licensed naturopathic medical doctor in private practice, Stengler Center for Integrative Medicine, Encinitas, California...author of many books, including *The Natural Physician's Healing Therapies* and coauthor of *Prescription for Natural Cures*.

Some of my patients who have type 2 diabetes are able to keep the disease under control with diet, exercise and supplements. Lucky them! But for other diabetes patients, that's not enough and they must take pharmaceutical medications.

I'm happy to report that there is another natural treatment option for diabetes patients who currently take pharmaceutical medications. Research has found that a plant extract called berberine can control diabetes as well as, or better than, common medications such as *metformin* (Glucophage) and *rosiglitazone* (Avandia). And it does this with no side effects—and without damaging the liver, as some medications do. *Here's how berberine can help people with diabetes…*

A naturally occurring chemical compound, berberine is found in the roots and stems of several plants, including *Hydrastis canadensis* (goldenseal), *Coptis chinensis* (coptis or goldthread) and Berberis aquifolium (Oregon grape). Long used as a remedy in Chinese and Ayurvedic medicines, berberine is known for its antimicrobial properties and as a treatment for bacterial and fungal infections. Several decades ago, berberine was used to treat diarrhea in patients in China. That was when doctors noticed that the blood sugar levels of diabetes patients were lower after taking the herbal extract—and berberine began to be investigated for this purpose.

Over the past 20 years, there has been much research on berberine and its effectiveness in treating diabetes. In 2008, Chinese researchers published a study in Metabolism in which adults with newly diagnosed type 2 diabetes were given 500 milligrams (mg) of either berberine or the drug metformin three times a day for three months. Researchers found that berberine did as good a job as metformin at regulating glucose metabolism, as indicated by hemoglobin A1C (a measure of blood glucose over several weeks)…fasting blood glucose…blood sugar after eating…and level of insulin after eating. Berberine even reduced the amount of insulin needed to turn glucose into energy by 45%! In addition, those taking berberine had noticeably lower trigylceride and total cholesterol levels than those taking metformin.

In another 2008 study published in J*ournal of Clinical Endocrinology and Metabolism*, researchers found that type 2 diabetes pa-

tients who were given berberine had significant reductions in fasting and postmeal blood glucose, hemoglobin A1C, triglycerides, total cholesterol and LDL (bad) cholesterol—and also lost an average of five pounds, to boot, during the three-month study period.

In a 2010 study in *Metabolism*, Chinese researchers compared people with type 2 diabetes who took either 1,000 mg daily of berberine or daily doses of metformin or rosiglitazone. After two months, berberine had lowered subjects' fasting blood glucose levels by an average of about 30%, an improvement over the rosiglitazone group and almost as much as people in the metformin group. Berberine also reduced subjects' hemoglobin A1C by 18%—equal to rosiglitazone and, again, almost as good as metformin. In addition, berberine lowered serum insulin levels by 28.2% (indicating increased insulin sensitivity)…lowered triglycerides by 17.5%…and actually improved liver enzyme levels. Pharmaceutical medications, on the other hand, have the potential to harm the liver.

These were remarkable findings. Here was a botanical that was holding up to scientific scrutiny—and performing as well as, or better than, some drugs that patients had been taking for diabetes for years.

HOW BERBERINE WORKS IN THE BODY

Berberine helps to lower blood glucose in several ways. One of its primary mechanisms involves stimulating the activity of the genes responsible for manufacturing and activating insulin receptors, which are critical for controlling blood glucose.

Berberine also has an effect on blood sugar regulation through activation of incretins, gastrointestinal hormones that affect the amount of insulin released by the body after eating.

HOW BERBERINE CAN HELP

I recommend berberine to my patients with newly diagnosed type 2 diabetes to reduce their blood sugar and prevent them from needing pharmaceutical drugs. When a diet, exercise and supplement program (including supplements such as chromium) is already helping a diabetes patient, I don't recommend that he/she switch to berberine.

Some patients are able to take berberine—and make dietary changes—and stop taking diabetes drugs altogether. People with severe diabetes can use berberine in conjunction with medication—and this combination treatment allows for fewer side effects and better blood sugar control. I don't recommend berberine for prediabetes unless diet and exercise are not effective. Berberine is sold in health-food stores and online in tablet and capsule form. The dosage I typically recommend for all diabetes patients is 500 mg twice daily.

For patients with diabetes who want to use berberine, I recommend talking to your doctor about taking this supplement. It's also important for every patient with diabetes to participate in a comprehensive diet and exercise program.

Note that berberine helps patients with type 2 diabetes, not type 1 diabetes (in which the body does not produce enough insulin).

The Secret Invasion That Causes Diabetes

George L. King, MD, research director and chief scientific officer of Harvard's Joslin Diabetes Center, where he heads the vascular cell biology research section, and professor of medicine at Harvard School of Public Health in Boston. Dr. King is coauthor, with Royce Flippin, of *The Diabetes Reset: Avoid It, Control It, Even Reverse It—A Doctor's Scientific Program.*

I t's easy to get the impression that diabetes is all about blood sugar. Most people with diabetes check their glucose levels at least once a day. Even people without diabetes are advised to have glucose tests every few years—just to make sure that the disease isn't creeping up on them.

But glucose is only part of the picture. Scientists now know that chronic inflammation increases the risk that you'll develop diabetes. If you already have insulin resistance (a precursor to diabetes) or full-blown diabetes, inflammation will make your glucose levels harder to manage.

A common mistake: Unfortunately, many doctors still don't test for inflammation even though it accompanies all of the main diabetes risk factors, including smoking, obesity and high-fat/sugar diets. *What you need to know about this important aspect of diabetes care…*

SILENT DAMAGE

You hear a lot about inflammation, but what exactly is it—and when is it a problem? Normal inflammation is protective. It comes on suddenly and lasts for just a few days or weeks—usually in response to an injury or infection. Inflammation kills or encapsulates microbes…assists in the formation of protective scar tissue…and helps regenerate damaged tissues.

But chronic inflammation—caused, for example, by infection or injuries that lead to continuously elevated levels of toxins—does not turn itself off. It persists for years or even decades, particularly in those who are obese, eat poor diets, don't get enough sleep or have chronic diseases, including seemingly minor conditions such as gum disease.

The diabetes link: Persistently high levels of inflammatory molecules interfere with the ability of insulin to regulate glucose—one cause of high blood sugar. Inflammation also appears to damage beta cells, the insulin-producing cells in the pancreas.

Studies have shown that when inflammation is aggressively lowered—with salsalate (an anti-inflammatory drug), for example—glucose levels can drop significantly. Inflammation is typically identified with a blood test that measures a marker known as CRP, or C-reactive protein (see below).

HOW TO FIGHT INFLAMMATION

Even though salsalate reduces inflammation, when taken in high doses, it causes too many side effects, such as stomach bleeding and ringing in the ears, to be used long term. *Safer ways to reduce inflammation and keep it down…*

•**Breathe clean air.** Smoke and smog threaten more than just your lungs. Recent research has shown that areas with the highest levels of airborne particulates that are small enough to penetrate deeply into the lungs have more than 20% higher rates of type 2 diabetes than areas with the lowest levels of these particulates.

Air pollution (including cigarette smoke) increases inflammation in fatty tissues and in the vascular system. In animal studies, exposure to air pollution increases both insulin resistance and the risk for full-fledged diabetes.

My advice: Most people—and especially those who live in polluted areas—could benefit from using an indoor HEPA filter or an electrostatic air filter.

Products such as the Honeywell Long-Life Pure HEPA QuietCare Air Purifier (available at Amazon.com for $97.41) will trap nearly 100% of harmful airborne particulates from indoor air.

If you live in a large metropolitan area, avoid outdoor exercise during high-traffic times of day.

●**Take care of your gums.** Even people who take good care of their teeth often neglect their gums. It's estimated that almost half of American adults have some degree of periodontal (gum) disease.

Why it matters: The immune system can't always eliminate infections that occur in gum pockets, the areas between the teeth and gums. A persistent gum infection causes equally persistent inflammation that contributes to other illnesses. For example, research shows that people with gum disease were twice as likely to develop diabetes as those without it.

My advice: After every meal (or at least twice a day), floss and brush, in that order. And clean your gums—gently use a soft brush. Twice a day, also use an antiseptic mouthwash (such as Listerine).

It's particularly important to follow these steps before you go to bed to remove bacteria that otherwise will remain undisturbed until morning.

●**Get more exercise.** It's among the best ways to control chronic inflammation because it burns fat. When you have less fat, you'll also produce fewer inflammation-promoting cytokines.

Data from the Nurses' Health Study and the Health Professionals Follow-Up Study found that walking briskly for a half hour daily re-

duced the risk of developing diabetes by nearly one-third.

My advice: Take 10,000 steps per day. To do this, walk whenever possible for daily activities, such as shopping, and even walk inside your home if you don't want to go out. Wear a pedometer to make sure you reach your daily goal.

●**Enjoy cocoa.** Cocoa contains a type of antioxidant known as flavanols, which have anti-inflammatory properties. Known primarily for their cardiovascular benefits, flavanols are now being found to help regulate insulin levels.

My advice: For inflammation-fighting effects, have one square of dark chocolate (with at least 70% cocoa) daily.

●**Try rose hip tea.** Rose hips are among the richest sources of vitamin C, with five times as much per cup than what is found in one orange. A type of rose hip known as rosa canina is particularly potent because it may contain an additional anti-inflammatory compound known as glycoside of mono and diglycerol (GOPO). It inhibits the production of a number of inflammatory molecules, including chemokines and interleukins.

My advice: Drink several cups of tangy rose hip tea a day. It's available both in bags and as a loose-leaf tea. If you're not a tea drinker, you can take rose hip supplements. Follow the directions on the label.

●**Season with turmeric.** This spice contains curcumin, one of the most potent anti-inflammatory agents. It inhibits the action of eicosanoids, "signaling molecules" that are involved in the inflammatory response.

My advice: Eat more turmeric—it's a standard spice in curries and yellow (not Dijon) mustard. You will want something more potent if you already have diabetes and/or elevated CRP. I often recommend Curamin, a potent form of curcumin that's combined with boswellia, another anti-inflammatory herb.

Important: Be sure to talk to your doctor before trying rose hip or turmeric supplements if you take medication or have a chronic health condition.

CHECK YOUR CRP LEVEL

An inexpensive and accurate blood test that is often used to estimate heart attack risk is also recommended for people who have diabetes or are at increased risk for it. The blood test measures C-reactive protein (CRP), a marker for inflammation, which can lead to heart disease and impair the body's ability to regulate glucose.

Doctors may recommend the test for patients beginning in their 30s. It's wise to get it earlier if you have diabetes risk factors, such as obesity or a family history.

A high-sensitivity CRP (hsCRP) test typically costs about $20 and is usually covered by insurance. A reading of less than 1 mg/L is ideal. Levels above 3 mg/L indicate a high risk for insulin resistance and diabetes as well as for heart attack.

If the first test shows that your CRP level is elevated, you'll want to do everything you can to lower it—for example, through exercise, a healthful diet and weight loss. Repeat the test every four to six months to see how well your lifestyle improvements are working.

To Prevent Diabetes, Say Hello to Your Kitchen

The path to diabetes prevention may lead to your stove, your oven and your pantry.

When researchers from Harvard's T.H. Chan School of Public Health analyzed data on nearly 100,000 men and women who were followed for up to 36 years, for each lunch eaten at home each week, the risk of developing diabetes went down 2%. For every weekly dinner, it dropped 4%. Those who ate 11 to 14 lunches or dinners at home each week compared with those who ate only six meals, for example, were 13% less likely to get diabetes.

Why? Many studies have found that home cooking tends to be lower in fat, sugar and calories than restaurant fare, especially fast food, so it's no surprise that the eat-at-home folks in the study weighed less than those who more

128

frequently ate out. They also drank fewer sugar-sweetened beverages.

Study by researchers at Harvard T.H. Chan School of Public Health, Boston, and Montefiore Medical Center, New York City, presented at the annual meeting of the American Heart Association.

Reverse Your Diabetes in Three Weeks!

Stefan Ripich, ND, a naturopathic physician based in Santa Fe, New Mexico. He practiced for 10 years at the Palo Alto Veterans Administration Medical Center and established the first holistic clinic in the VA system.

In the US, a new case of diabetes is diagnosed every 30 seconds. And many of those people will be given drugs to treat the disease.

You can control high blood sugar with medications, but they aren't a cure and they can have side effects. They also are expensive, costing $400 or more a month for many patients.

Much better: Dietary remedies that have been proven to reduce blood sugar, improve the effects of insulin (a hormone produced by the pancreas that controls blood sugar), promote weight loss and, in many cases, eliminate the need for medications. A UCLA study found that 50% of patients with type 2 diabetes (the most common form) were able to reverse it in three weeks with dietary changes and exercise.

How you can do it, too…

•**Eliminate all HFCS.** A 2010 Princeton study found that rats given water sweetened with high-fructose corn syrup (HFCS) gained more weight than rats that drank water sweetened with plain sugar, even though their calorie intake was exactly the same.

Reasons: The calories from HFCS fail to trigger leptin, the hormone that tells your body when to quit eating. Also, HFCS is more likely than natural sugar to be converted to fat… and being overweight is the main risk factor for diabetes.

What to do: Read food labels carefully. HFCS is the main sweetener in soft drinks and many processed foods, including baked goods such as cookies and cakes.

• **Don't drink diet soda.** If you give up HFCS-laden soft drinks, don't switch to diet soda. Diet sodas actually cause weight gain by boosting insulin production, leading to excessively high insulin in your blood that triggers greater fat accumulation and even more cravings for sugar. A study published in *Diabetes Care* found that drinking diet soda every day increased the risk for type 2 diabetes by as much as 67%. If you crave sweet bubbly beverages, pour one inch of pure fruit juice into a glass and then top it off with carbonated water.

• **Eat barley.** I advise patients to eat foods that are as close to their natural state as possible —whole-grain cereals and breads, brown rice, etc. These "slow carbohydrates" contain fiber and other substances that prevent the spikes in glucose and insulin that lead to diabetes.

Best choice: Barley. Researchers at the Creighton Diabetes Center in Omaha compared the effects of two breakfasts—one consisting of oatmeal (one of the best slow carbohydrates) and the other consisting of an even slower breakfast cereal made from barley. Participants who ate barley had a postmeal rise in blood sugar that was significantly lower than participants who ate the oatmeal breakfast. You can eat cooked barley as a side dish…sprinkle it on salads…or mix it into tuna, chicken, tofu or lentil salad.

• **Season with cinnamon.** About one-quarter teaspoon of cinnamon daily reduces blood sugar, improves insulin sensitivity and reduces inflammation in the arteries—important for reducing the risk for heart disease, the leading cause of death in diabetics. Research published in *Diabetes Care* found that people with type 2 diabetes who ate at least one-quarter teaspoon of cinnamon daily reduced fasting blood sugar levels by up to 29%. They also had up to a 30% reduction in triglycerides (a blood fat) and up to a 27% drop in LDL (bad) cholesterol.

• **Eat protein at breakfast.** Protein at breakfast stabilizes blood sugar and makes people feel satisfied, which means that you'll consume fewer calories overall. Lean protein includes eggs, chicken and fish.

• **Eat more meat (the good kind).** We've all been told that a diet high in meat (and therefore saturated fat) is inherently unhealthy. Not true. Other things being equal, people who eat more saturated fat actually tend to weigh less and have smaller waist measurements than similar adults who eat less. The real danger is from processed meats, such as bacon, hot dogs and many cold cuts. These foods have more calories per serving than natural meats. They're higher in sodium. They have a lower percentage of heart-healthy omega-3 fatty acids and other beneficial fats that lower inflammation. A large study that looked at data from 70,000 women found that those who ate processed meats with every meal were 52% more likely to develop diabetes than those who ate healthier meats and other foods.

I advise people to look for grass-fed beef. It's lower in calories and fat than industrialized grain-fed factory feedlot beef and higher in omega-3s.

• **Snack on nuts.** Healthful snacking between meals keeps blood sugar stable throughout the day. Nuts are the perfect snack because they're high in fiber (which reduces abrupt increases in glucose and insulin) and protein (for appetite control). They also are good sources of important nutrients and antioxidants. A Harvard study of 83,000 women found that those who frequently ate almonds, pecans or other nuts were 27% less likely to develop diabetes than those who rarely ate nuts. A small handful every day is enough.

Caution: "Roasted" nuts usually are a bad choice because they often are deep-fried in coconut oil. They also have added salt and/or sugar. "Dry-roasted nuts" have not been fried in fat but usually have salt and sugar.

If you like roasted nuts, it's best to buy organically grown raw nuts and lightly toast them in a dry fry pan over very low heat (or in your oven).

• **Supplement with vitamin D.** In theory, we can get all the vitamin D that we need from sunshine—our bodies make it after the sun hits our skin. But about 90% of Americans don't get adequate amounts—either because they deliberately avoid sun exposure or because they live in climates without much sun. A Finnish study found that participants with high levels of vitamin D were 40% less likely to develop diabetes than those with lower amounts. Vitamin D appears to improve insulin sensitivity and reduce the risk for diabetes-related complications, including heart disease.

Recommended: Take 1,000 international units (IU) to 2,000 IU of vitamin D-3 daily.

•**Remember to exercise.** It's just as important as a healthy diet for preventing and reversing diabetes. The Diabetes Prevention Program (a major multicenter clinical research study) found that people who walked as little as 17 minutes a day, on average, were 58% less likely to develop diabetes. Walking for 30 minutes most days of the week is optimal.

Walnuts May Cut Diabetes Risk

Women who ate at least eight ounces of walnuts a month were 24% less likely to develop type 2 diabetes than women who ate none, in a recent finding.

Possible reason: Walnuts are especially rich in polyunsaturated fats, which may help prevent diabetes. They also have high amounts of dietary fiber, antioxidants and other beneficial substances. The results most likely apply to men, too.

Frank Hu, MD, PhD, professor of nutrition and epidemiology, Harvard School of Public Health, and professor of medicine, Harvard Medical School, both in Boston. He is senior author of a study published in *Journal of Nutrition.*

Popular Drinks That Decrease Risk for Diabetes 25%

Coffee and tea lower diabetes risk. People who drank three or more cups of coffee daily had a 25% lower risk for type 2 diabetes than people who drank two or fewer cups. Similar results were shown for tea and decaffeinated coffee, indicating that the effect is not entirely due to caffeine but is likely to include other compounds present in these beverages, such as magnesium.

Rachel Huxley, DPhil, director of the nutrition and lifestyle division and associate professor in the faculty of medicine, University of Sydney, Australia, and lead author of a meta-analysis of 18 studies involving more than 450,000 people, published in *Archives of Internal Medicine.*

9

Have the Best Sex of Your Life After 60!

A Couple's Guide to Boosting Desire

One out of five marriages is virtually sexless—these couples have sex 10 or fewer times a year. In about one in three marriages, one spouse has a considerably larger sexual appetite than the other. If you see yourself in these statistics, don't despair—there's a great deal that can be done to boost your marriage's libido.

WHO'S SEX-STARVED?

A sex-starved marriage occurs when one spouse is desperately longing for more physical affection. Sex-starved marriages can't be defined by the number of times per week or month that a couple has sex, because there are no daily or weekly minimum requirements to ensure a healthy sex life. What works for one couple is grounds for divorce for another.

Most people believe that it is principally women who struggle with low sexual desire. While it's true that more men than women complain about the frequency of sex, the difference between genders isn't great. In fact, low desire in men is one of America's best-kept secrets. Too many men are simply unwilling to discuss their low desire with doctors, therapists or even their wives.

In a sex-starved marriage, the less interested spouse, whether male or female, typically thinks, Why are you making such a big deal out of this? It's just sex. But to the spouse wanting more physical closeness, sex is extremely important because it's not just a physical act. It's about feeling wanted, attractive, appreciated and emotionally connected. When the low-desire spouse doesn't understand sex's significance and continues to reject sexual advances, intimacy on many different levels tends to fall off. The couple stops cuddling on the couch, laughing at each other's jokes, going on dates together. In short, they

---

Michele Weiner-Davis, MSW, social worker and relationship expert who is founder and director of the Divorce Busting Center in Boulder, Colorado. She is author of seven books, including, *The Sex-Starved Wife: What to Do When He's Lost Desire*. Divorcebusting.com

131

stop being friends. This places their marriage in jeopardy.

CATCH-22

Frequently, the lower-desire spouse needs to feel close and connected on an emotional level before he/she is interested in being sexual. This usually entails spending quality time together and talking about intimate issues.

The catch-22 is that typically the higher-desire spouse needs to feel connected physically in order to open up with conversation or feel that spending time together is a priority.

One spouse waits for time together and heart-to-heart talks before investing in the physical relationship, while the other spouse waits to be touched before initiating time together or intimate conversation.

Each waits for the other to change.

THE NOs HAVE VETO POWER

The spouse with the lower sexual drive usually controls the frequency of sex—if he or she doesn't want it, it generally doesn't happen. This is not due to maliciousness or a desire for power—it just seems unimaginable to be sexual if one partner is not in the mood.

Furthermore, there is an unspoken and often unconscious expectation that the higher-desire spouse must accept the no-sex verdict, not complain about it—and, of course, remain monogamous. After decades of working with couples, I can attest that this is an unfair and unworkable arrangement. This is not to say that infidelity is a solution, but as with all relationship conflicts, being willing to find middle ground is the best way to ensure love's longevity.

If you're in a sex-starved marriage, you and your spouse need to make some changes. Don't worry about who takes the lead. Relationships are such that if one person changes, the relationship changes.

ADVICE FOR HIGH-DESIRE SPOUSES

Tune in to your spouse's needs outside the bedroom. High-desire people usually try to boost their spouses' desire by doing things that would turn themselves on, such as buying sexy lingerie and renting X-rated videos. However, these actions often don't work for their spouses, who are more likely to be responsive to loving behaviors outside the bedroom, such

as helping more with housework and offering more compliments and fewer criticisms.

• **Talk from the heart.** Some people talk to their spouses about their sexual unhappiness, but instead of speaking from their hearts—which might prompt their spouses' empathy—harsh words are exchanged and tempers flare. Although it's understandable that unending rejection might lead to anger and resentment, these emotions are not aphrodisiacs. Instead of complaining, say, "I miss being close to you physically. We seem to get along so much better after we make love. I'm hoping that we can be more affectionate this week."

ADVICE FOR LOW-DESIRE SPOUSES

• **Don't ignore the problem.** If you and your spouse have been arguing about sex, don't stick your head in the sand. Your differences won't disappear—the only thing that will disappear is your intimate connection and friendship. There are many excellent resources to help you feel more sexual. Good books include *Hot Monogamy* by Patricia Love, MD, and Jo Robinson...*Rekindling Desire: A Step-by-Step Program to Help Low-Sex and No-Sex Marriages* by Barry and Emily McCarthy...and my book, *The Sex-Starved Marriage.* Also, licensed sex therapists can be found through the American Association of Sexuality Educators, Counselors and Therapists (*www.aasect.org*).

• **Just do it.** Perhaps you've had the experience of not being in the mood when your spouse approached you, but you gave it a try, and once you got into it, you enjoyed it. You're not alone. There are millions of people who simply don't experience out-of-the-blue sexy thoughts—unlike their more highly sexed spouses who may have lusty thoughts many times every day.

Try this: For the next two weeks, initiate sex twice each week. Also, flirt, call your spouse pet names, dress more provocatively and be more physically affectionate. Do this whether you feel like it or not. Then carefully watch your spouse for any changes in his behavior. An irritable, withdrawn, uncooperative spouse most likely will become much more fun to be around.

Super Sex Every Time: Natural Cures for Impotence, Low Desire, Dryness, More

Brigitte Mars, herbalist, a founding member of The American Herbalists Guild and instructor at Naropa University, Bauman College and Boulder College of Massage Therapy, all in Boulder, Colorado. She has been practicing and teaching herbal medicine and nutrition for more than 40 years. She is author of *The Sexual Herbal: Prescriptions for Enhancing Love and Passion.* BrigitteMars.com

Couples who enjoy sex regularly tend to live longer than those who rarely or never have sex.

Yet millions of Americans struggle to have satisfying sex, or any sex, because of physical limitations. Medications can help with problems such as an inability to get erections or vaginal dryness, but they don't always work—and can carry the risk for side effects.

Better: Natural remedies that improve energy and libido as well as sexual performance. In my 40 years of specializing in herbal medicine, I have found them to be quite effective for many people. (The herbs and supplements noted here are readily available at most health-food stores and online.)

LUBRICATION

Vaginal dryness can be as problematic for a woman as erectile dysfunction is for a man. Women naturally produce less moisture (in the vagina, as well as in the eyes, skin and other parts of the body) as they get older. But it's one of the easiest sexual problems to correct—and without the use of store-bought, chemical-filled lubricants. Try one of the following remedies. If that doesn't work, try another until you find what works best for you.

• **Barley water.** Barley water is an emollient that also nourishes and strengthens vaginal tissues. Cook two cups of light pearled barley in 10 cups of water for two hours. Strain, and reserve the water. Drink a glassful three or four times a day between meals for at least three weeks. If it helps, continue doing it. It can be kept in the refrigerator for up to three days. (You can use the leftover barley in soups and salads.)

• **Acidophilus.** Dryness is sometimes caused by an overgrowth of vaginal yeast. Before going to bed each night, insert a capsule of acidophilus into the vagina. It inhibits yeast and helps the vagina produce more lubrication.

Important: Don't use an enteric-coated capsule—it won't dissolve readily. Use an acidophilus gel capsule.

• **Chemical-free lubricant.** Mix one ounce of softened cocoa butter with one tablespoon each of powdered dong quai (an herb in the parsley family), licorice root and marshmallow root, along with one tablespoon of powdered wild yam and two tablespoons of vitamin E oil.

Optional: Two drops of essential oil of rose for a pleasant aroma.

Roll the mixture into suppository shapes about the size of your little finger. Store them in a glass jar in the refrigerator for up to six months. Insert one in the vagina daily before bedtime.

LOW LIBIDO

If your sex drive is lower than you (or your partner) would like…

• **Eat black foods.** According to Traditional Chinese Medicine, the kidneys govern sexual vitality. Foods with natural black color, such as black olives, black sesame seeds, chia seeds and black beans, strengthen the kidneys and improve sexual energy and performance.

Bonus: Black olives and chia increase the production of mucilage, important for sexual lubrication.

• **Muira puama.** This is a South American herb that traditionally is used as an aphrodisiac and to improve erections as well as orgasms in men and women. It's a warming herb that increases circulation. If you have cold hands and/or feet, you probably have impaired circulation to the genitals as well. Muira puama can help.

Dose: One-half cup of muira puama tea…or 10 to 30 drops of tincture, mixed with an inch of water or taken straight, three times daily. Also available in capsules. Natives of South America sometimes apply the cooled tea directly to the genitals as a sexual stimulant.

133

- **DHEA,** an over-the-counter hormonal supplement that's converted to testosterone in the body, can increase libido and sexual responsiveness in women and men.

Important: Improper dosing can cause acne, the growth of facial hair in women and other side effects—including an increased risk for some cancers. Take DHEA only under the supervision of a doctor.

ERECTILE DYSFUNCTION

The arteries that carry blood to the penis are just slightly wider than the head of a pin. Even slight buildups of plaque (atherosclerosis) can impede circulation and make it difficult for a man to get and/or maintain an erection.

The same things that improve overall cardiovascular health, such as lowering cholesterol and blood pressure, can improve a man's ability to achieve an erection. *Also helpful…*

- **The Deer.** This is a Taoist exercise that removes energy blockages, stimulates hormone production and improves erections. Sit on the edge of the bed, and rub your hands to warm them. Hold the scrotum with one hand. With the other hand, massage right below the navel in a circular motion. Do it 81 times, then switch hands and rub in the other direction 81 times.

Follow this with 36 Kegel exercises, in which you tighten and then release the pubococcygeus muscles—the same muscles that you would use to stop urine in midstream.

- **Foot massage.** Once or twice a day, massage the entire foot, paying particular attention to the sides of the heels. The meridians (energy pathways) that support sexual potency run through this part of the foot.

- **Yohimbe.** Yohimbe bark extract is among the most effective natural products for improving erections. It increases blood flow to the genitals while at the same time impeding the flow of blood out of the penis—important for keeping an erection.

Dose: One cup of yohimbe tea…or 30 drops of tincture, mixed with an inch of water or taken straight, 30 minutes to an hour before sex. Also available in capsules.

Caution: Yohimbe can elevate blood pressure and cause insomnia. It also interacts with many common drugs, including antihypertensives and heart and diabetes medications. Use it only under the supervision of a doctor and never more than twice a week.

- **Omega-3 fatty acids enhance circulation and help the nervous system function better.** Eat fish (such as salmon, tuna, sardines) twice per week or supplement with fish oil (follow directions on the label).

BETTER ORGASMS

Women (and men) who eat well, exercise regularly and are comfortable with their bodies experience better and more frequent orgasms. *Also helpful…*

- **Arginine.** An amino acid called L-arginine is a vasodilator, which means it helps to widen or open up blood vessels. Arginine cream can be applied to the clitoris (or to the penis) before sex to increase arousal and the intensity of orgasms. You also can take an oral capsule form to increase blood flow to sexual organs. Follow directions on the label.

Sleeping in the Buff...

Michael Breus, PhD, sleep specialist in private practice in Scottsdale, Arizona. SecretstoSleepSuccess.com

My husband likes to sleep in the nude, even on frigid winter nights. Should he put on some pajamas?

Not necessarily. There are many health benefits to sleeping naked (but it is inadvisable with small children around or pets in the bed). New research has found that sleeping in a chilly room (or staying cool by sleeping naked) increases brown fat, a healthy type of fat that burns calories to make heat. For the best night's sleep, aim for a bedroom temperature of about 65°F and keep your hands and feet warm.

Men (and women) who sleep in their underwear or tight pajamas are more likely to get genital infections due to trapped heat and moisture. But the best benefit of sleeping in the nude may be skin-to-skin contact between bed partners, which triggers the release of the feel-good hormone oxytocin. Studies have shown that oxytocin increases a feeling of connection between partners, relieves stress and lowers blood pressure. So why not shed your winter PJs and join him?

How Women Can Feel Sexier Again (Without Popping a Pill)

Kathryn Hall, PhD, a licensed psychologist and sex therapist with a private practice in Princeton, New Jersey. She is president-elect of the Society for Sex Therapy and Research, and author of *Reclaiming Your Sexual Self: How You Can Bring Desire Back Into Your Life*. DrKathrynHall.com

If you're a woman, everyone wants to help you with your sex drive.

The medical profession may classify you as having hypoactive sexual desire disorder (HSDD)…aka, low libido. The drug industry wants to sell you its latest pill.

The good news: If low sex drive bothers you, there are better ways than popping a pill to rekindle the flames of desire.

BEYOND THE LITTLE PINK PILL

The pharmaceutical industry is excited about *flibanserin* (Addyi), the first-ever drug approved for low libido in women, but many doctors and mental health professionals aren't so jazzed about it. It doesn't move the desire needle much, and there are worrisome side effects. And did we mention that you're supposed to take it every day…but you can't take it if you drink alcohol? To learn more, see Bottom Line's 12 Things You Should Know About the New Female Viagra.

Even the HSDD diagnosis itself is controversial. "There is no evidence that hypoactive sexual desire disorder is a medical condition," according a report in *Journal of Medical Ethics*. The author documents the extensive marketing campaign that the pharmaceutical industry sponsored to convince physicians that HSDD is, in fact, real—and thus needs to be treated with a drug.

Still, there's no question that many women do struggle with a lack of desire, and that it can

have real, sometimes painful, effects on their sense of well-being, as well as on their relationships. If you're dealing with lagging libido—and you can't or don't want to try the new "little pink pill"—what can you do about it?

To find out, we spoke with noted sex therapist Kathryn Hall, PhD, a psychologist in Princeton, New Jersey.

LOW LIBIDO IS VERY COMMON AND VERY NORMAL

There are many, many reasons why women lose desire for sex—relationship problems, stress, fatigue, body image issues, hormonal changes in menopause, medications such as anti-depressants, as well as depression itself, Dr. Hall noted. But you don't have to have a reason. Many women don't. *Here's why…*

It's very common for women to lose sexual desire as a relationship progresses over time from lust to love.

"We know from a lot of studies that for many women, desire—their spontaneous lust—seems to wane in midlife," Dr. Hall says. "It's a normal pattern to lose that sort of lustful feeling, and it doesn't mean there's something wrong with you." The truth is, there's no "normal" when it comes to desire and how it plays out. If you don't want to have sex very often, or at all, and that doesn't bother you or your partner (if you have one), that's fine. Your desire, or lack thereof, is only a concern if it's distressing for you or problematic for your relationship.

If it does bother you, on the other hand, Dr. Hall has some suggestions that she's seen work for the many couples she's counseled. *Here they are…*

REKINDLING DESIRE

For women, what often replaces lust is "responsive desire"—getting in the mood after things have already gotten going because her partner has taken the initiative. That's perfectly fine for many couples. But some partners may resent always having to initiate sex. And many women miss the excitement of lust and eventually start to feel like sex is an obligatory chore, something they have to do so their significant others don't get angry. Fortunately, Dr. Hall has seen many patients and couples work with these challenges to improve their sex lives, although she acknowledges that it's not necessarily an easy road. *Here are some of the strategies she believes can help...*

• **Be realistic about sex, but don't give up on it.** Now that you know that a lot of women struggle with a low sex drive, you can work on bringing desire back into your life. "You've made a decision that you need sex in your life and in your relationship and that you're going to put some energy and effort into it," Dr. Hall says. "It's not going to happen naturally." And that's OK.

• **Have maintenance sex.** "A lot of couples who stay sexual throughout their life span have what I call 'maintenance sex,'" Dr. Hall says. They think, "OK, it has been a while and I don't really feel like it but, you know what? I'm going to put some effort into it because we need sex in our life and in our relationship." Hall says these couples understand that bad sex happens and boring sex happens, but they still make lovemaking a priority because most of the time sex is satisfying.

• **Set yourself up for success.** The first step is to get out of the rut of feeling that sex is a chore. Start by challenging the belief that you never want to have sex with your partner. Think about the occasions when you enjoy it more, such as when you've just shared a nice time doing something together, and choose those kinds of situations for initiating sex—rather than if it's late and you have to get up early and go to work the next morning, or when you've been fighting.

• **Reengage with your own desire.** You may feel like you want to get sex over as quickly as possible. For many women, that means focusing only on satisfying their partners to get the deed done. Hurry up. You don't need to take care of me. Let's just focus on you. Have your orgasm and then we'll be done. If this sounds like your internal dialogue during sex, try slowing down and paying attention to what you need and want sexually. Put on some clothing that makes you feel sexy. Watch some erotica or, if you've ever used one, get your vibrator out. Have a glass of wine if that helps. Do these things not because you think it's going to turn your partner on, but because it's going to turn you on. And don't forget to

clue your partner into what you like. He or she is probably dying to know!

• **Make an effort to initiate sex.** This is probably the furthest thing from your mind, but it may be a big deal to your partner. Dr. Hall says: "When couples come in to see me, the man will often say, 'Look, I'm always the one that initiates this, and I don't like doing that. I want to be desired.' Of course he does, right? Men in their midlife want to feel like, 'Hey, I'm still vital and attractive and desirable,' and, if his partner never wants to initiate sex with him, it doesn't feel great." Being more mindful about initiating sex from time to time can go a long way toward making your partner feel physically cherished—and that can only reap benefits for you.

Feeding Your Libido-Boosting Hormones

Michael Aziz, MD, is founder and director of Midtown Integrative Medicine and a board-certified internist at Lenox Hill Hospital, both in New York City. He also is the author of *The Perfect 10 Diet: 10 Key Hormones That Hold the Secret to Losing Weight and Feeling Great—Fast!* Perfect10diet.com

---

If your sex life has been a bit sluggish of late, the problem may lie in the kitchen, not the bedroom.

Reason: The foods you eat affect—for better or worse—your body's production of the hormones needed for a healthy libido and the hormones that dampen desire.

Specific foods that can stimulate or sap a woman's sex drive. He told me that a libido-boosting diet is not a quick fix because there is no scientific proof that eating a particular food just prior to sex can spark arousal. Rather, the idea is to adopt a healthy lifestyle—including a hormone-optimizing diet—to improve your sex life.

Libido is affected by many things, of course, including your relationship with your partner, your emotional state, stress level, sleep quality and overall health. But regardless of these, if you make certain changes to your diet, you are taking a valuable step toward improving your sex life.

Are you ready to ensure that your desire for sex and ability to enjoy it are functioning at their best? *Here's what you need to know...*

The older we get, the more helpful the right diet can be in keeping our sex drive alive. Estrogen and progesterone, the female hormones that promote sexual desire, deplete naturally with age. So does testosterone, which plays a crucial role in women's libido even though it is known as a 'male' sex hormone. But sex hormones don't tell the whole story, because growth and stress hormones also affect sexual desire. And all of these are influenced by what you eat.

There's no exact prescription for the "right" amount of a particular libido-enhancing nutrient. No one can promise you, "Eat two oysters every day and you'll be frisky every night." Instead, your goal is for your diet to incorporate moderate-to-ample amounts of the nutrients needed for optimal hormonal balance.

Be sure that your diet includes...

•**Natural fats.** We have had it drilled into our heads that we should severely restrict all fats to reduce heart disease risk and maintain a healthy weight—but to produce sex hormones, the body needs some saturated and monounsaturated fats. Natural hormone-balancing fats are found in avocados, butter, fish, nuts, olive oil and whole milk.

•**Cholesterol-rich foods.** Here is another group that seems counterintuitive, but the type of cholesterol found in foods is not the same as the type that clogs arteries. Actually, dietary cholesterol aids in the production of sex hormones—so include moderate amounts of eggs, liver, organic red meats and shellfish in your diet.

•**Omega-3 fatty acids.** You know that these protect against heart disease...but did you know that what's good for your heart is also good for your genitals?

Reason: Omega-3s improve blood flow, and the more blood that reaches the genitals, the more aroused you feel. From a hormonal standpoint, omega-3s optimize female sex hormone production...and as a bonus, they help maintain the moisture and health of vaginal tissues. Good sources include fatty fish (halibut, mackerel, salmon, sardines, tuna) as well as eggs, flaxseed oil and walnuts.

•**Zinc.** This mineral is essential to support the production of female and male sex hormones. Oysters are particularly rich in zinc...clams, crabs, lobster and shrimp are good sources, too. Zinc also is found in barley, buckwheat, cheese, chickpeas, nuts (almonds, cashews, peanuts, walnuts), oat bran, poultry, red meat, seeds (pumpkin, squash, sunflower) and spinach.

•**Citrulline.** This amino acid converts to arginine, a substance that dilates blood vessels, and thus improves blood flow ("like a natural Viagra). Citrulline is abundant in watermelon...it also is found in cantaloupe, cucumbers and milk.

Limit these libido killers...

•**Sugar.** Eating sweets triggers production of the stress hormone cortisol. This interferes with arousal because, to create that cortisol, the body uses up some of the sex hormone progesterone. Sugar also impairs production of the steroid hormone DHEA, a precursor the body uses to create sex hormones.

•**Alcohol.** A drink can increase desire by lowering inhibitions—but it also shuts down sex hormones. If you do drink, limit yourself to no more than three servings per week.

•**Manufactured fats.** Trans fats—such as those in margarine, hydrogenated oils and vegetable shortening—damage DHEA and interfere with production of female and male sex hormones.

•**Caffeine.** In addition to breaking down testosterone, excessive caffeine can disrupt production of human growth hormone (HGH)—and HGH is the closest thing we have to a fountain of youth.

Best: Limit caffeine intake to no more than two servings per day to help keep your libido lively.

Sex After a Long Dry Spell

Barbara Bartlik, MD, is a sex therapist and assistant clinical professor of psychiatry at Weill Cornell Medical College in New York City. She is the author of numerous scientific publications and medical advisor for the book *Extraordinary Togetherness: A Woman's Guide to Love, Sex and Intimacy.*

When you haven't been intimate for years, intercourse is likely to be uncomfortable at first because the vagina can atrophy from lack of activity. Also, if you are postmenopausal, vaginal tissues can become thin and dry due to the natural decline in estrogen and testosterone levels, exacerbating the discomfort of penetration. Fortunately, there is a lot you can do now to prepare yourself so that intercourse will be enjoyable. *Try any or all of the following...*

•**Start using a nonhormonal over-the-counter vaginal moisturizer,** which is a topical suppository, cream or gel with long-lasting effects. Routinely applied two or three times per week, it helps rejuvenate the vaginal tissues, making them more moist and resilient.

Good brand: Replens.

•**Once daily, use a pin to pierce a vitamin E gel-cap supplement (500 IU),** squeeze the oil onto your fingertips, then rub it onto the labia and around the vaginal opening. This plumps up and strengthens the cells.

•**Ask your gynecologist whether a prescription topical estrogen cream or suppository is appropriate for you.** Topical estrogen can improve the integrity of the vaginal lining, reducing the chances of tearing and lessening any discomfort you might experience during sex—and because very little gets into the bloodstream, it does not carry the same level of risk for systemic side effects as oral estrogen does. (Topical estrogen generally is not recommended for women at high risk for breast or ovarian cancer, but there are exceptions.) Also ask about specially compounded testosterone cream to be applied to the vulva. Though not FDA-approved for this purpose, doctors have been prescribing this to women for many years.

•**Keep a water-based or silicone-based personal lubricant on hand so you'll have it when you need it.** Used during foreplay and intercourse, it helps minimize pain and heighten pleasure. Some lubricants contain ingredients that can irritate delicate tissues, particularly in menopausal women, so look for a product that is organic, hypoallergenic and/or paraben-free.

Excellent brands include: Hathor Aphrodisia, Pink and Sliquid.

•**Do Kegel exercises, aiming for 20 minutes or 200 repetitions per day.** Repeatedly squeezing and then releasing the muscles you use to start and stop the flow of urine can increase the flow of blood, oxygen and nutrients to the pelvic floor, strengthening not only the muscles but also the tissues in that area.

Bonus: Kegels help prevent incontinence and may intensify orgasms.

•**Masturbate on your own, with a vibrator if desired, to rediscover what makes you feel aroused.** Sometimes getting back in the game takes practice.

•**Consider talking to your gynecologist about a vaginal dilator,** which is a set of smooth cylindrical probes in varying sizes. You use the dilator at home to gradually stretch the vagina—so that by the time you want to have intercourse, you are physically ready.

How to Stay Together Forever: Advice from Couples Who Split Up

Adrienne Jackson, PhD, assistant professor in the division of physical therapy, Florida Agricultural and Mechanical University, Tallahassee.

If you want your marriage to succeed, it pays to know why other marriages fail. I have tracked 373 married couples for the past 26 years as part of a study funded by the National Institutes of Health. The goal was to investigate how marriages really work over the long term—but many marriages don't work, at least not forever. Of those 373 couples, 46% have divorced, roughly in line with national averages.

What went wrong in those failed marriages? And what would those divorced people do differently if they could start over again? When I put those questions to my study participants, key trends emerged.

Surprising: Sex was not a major issue when it came to what divorced people said they would "change" if they could start over again. And it wasn't a key predictor of divorce over time in my study.

EXPAND CONVERSATIONS

Divorced people typically report that a lack of communication wasn't the problem in their relationships—they spoke with their spouses often during their marriages. But when these divorced people considered the content of their conversations, many admitted that the vast majority were about the business of the household—what chores needed to get done, what time they would be returning home from work, whether they were running low on peanut butter. Such conversations are necessary in a marriage, but they do little to make couples feel close.

What to do: Discuss your goals and dreams regularly with your partner, and encourage your partner to do the same with you. Do this even if you've been married for years and already know quite well what your spouse wants out of life. Even if very little new information is supplied, having these conversations increases the odds that you and your spouse will continue to see each other as partners in your pursuit of your goals and dreams.

On days when you don't chat about big things such as goals and dreams, at least have conversations about topics you both enjoy talking about. These might include books, movies or current events—anything you both appreciate that's unrelated to your responsibilities and your marriage.

EXPRESS YOUR LOVE DAILY

Many of the divorced people in my study admitted that their partners often got pushed to the back burner when life became busy. Their spouses wound up feeling taken for granted—a feeling that can lead to divorce when it is allowed to persist.

What to do: Make a gesture that shows your love and makes your spouse feel special every day. These gestures can be quite simple. Take your spouse's hand and say, "I love you," or "Thank you for being a great husband/wife." Provide a kiss or hug at an unexpected moment. Or do a little thing that makes your spouse's life easier without being asked, such as bringing in the newspaper or starting the coffee in the morning. It isn't the size of the gestures that prevents spouses from feeling taken for granted. It's the consistency with which these gestures are made—once a day at a minimum.

Warning: Some people believe that wives care more about receiving gestures of love than husbands. In fact, divorce is particularly likely when husbands fail to receive these gestures. This probably is because married women tend to receive gestures of love from their friends and relations in addition to their husbands. Husbands typically receive them only from their wives, so they miss them even more when their wives don't provide them.

TALK MORE ABOUT MONEY

Many married couples don't talk about money any more than necessary. Finances are the number-one source of conflict in marriage, so avoiding this topic can seem like a good way to avoid stirring up trouble. But my research shows that talking less about money actually increases the odds of divorce. True, talks about money can trigger spats—but couples who avoid money talks increase the risk that their money issues will remain unresolved and escalate until they endanger the marriage.

Example: If a relationship's lines of communication about finances are closed, one partner might spend freely, not realizing that the other is becoming angrier and angrier about the couple's inability to save for retirement.

What to do: First, consider what money means to you. Does it represent security? Status? Love? Success as a provider? Think about how your parents handled finances, too, and whether that might be affecting your financial beliefs and behavior. Also, reflect upon your financial goals and priorities.

Next, have a few chats with your spouse about noninflammatory money-related topics, such as money you've managed to save or upcoming expenses that you both agree upon. Mixing in some low-stress money talks can prevent anxiety levels from skyrocketing every time money is mentioned.

After you've had a few painless money conversations, share your financial goals and priorities with your spouse, as well as any thoughts you have about what money means to you. Ask your partner to do the same, then try to find common ground with your spouse about family spending rules and limits.

Example: Agree to consult with each other on all purchases over a certain dollar amount.

BLAME "US" FOR PROBLEMS

When one or both spouses chronically blame the other for the marriage's problems, the result tends to be escalating anger. When one or both spouses chronically blame himself or herself for the marriage's problems, the result tends to be feelings of guilt or depression. In either case, the odds of divorce increase.

What to do: When you have a fight, try to blame the relationship or circumstances, not your spouse or yourself. Say things such as, "We were both tired when we said those things"…or "We just weren't communicating well."

Also, people who already have divorced should take care to not blame their former spouses or themselves for the failure of that marriage. Use phrases that absolve you both such as, "We married too young"…or "We just weren't compatible." Divorced people who persist in blaming their exes or themselves are more likely to struggle in future relationships as well.

DON'T LET BOREDOM LINGER

All long-term relationships go through ruts when nothing new happens. If those ruts are allowed to persist for years, the result can be boredom—and boredom increases the odds of divorce.

What to do: Inject passion and excitement into your marriage. *Three potential ways to do that…*

• **Add a new shared activity.** Take a new class together or travel together to an unfamiliar location. Doing new things together mimics the feelings of adventure and passion that you

experienced back in the exciting early days of the relationship.

• **Add mystery and surprise.** Leave a love note for your spouse in an unexpected place or plan a weekend getaway for the two of you without telling your partner where you're going.

• **Add adrenaline.** Ride a roller coaster together…see a scary movie together…or exercise together. Anything that gets your heart racing and adrenaline pumping will release chemicals into your brain similar to those experienced by people who are passionately in love. Do such things together with your spouse a few times, and these chemicals could help rekindle your passion, excitement and sexual arousal for each other.

Tasty Aphrodisiac

Women who drank red wine in moderation had more sexual interest and lubrication than ones who drank little or none.

Possible reason: The antioxidants and alcohol in the wine may increase production of nitric oxide, a gas that helps artery walls relax—increasing blood flow to genitals.

Caution: Drink no more than one to two glasses of red wine a day—any more decreases sexual response.

Study of 798 women by researchers at University of Florence, Italy, published in *The Journal of Sexual Medicine*.

Women: Increase Your Sex Drive Naturally

Laurie Steelsmith, ND, LAc, a licensed naturopathic physician and acupuncturist with a 20-year private practice in Honolulu. Dr. Steelsmith is coauthor of *Great Sex, Naturally: Every Woman's Guide to Enhancing Her Sexuality Through the Secrets of Natural Medicine.* DrLaurieSteelsmith.com

Diminished libido—little or no sexual desire—is the most common sexual complaint among women. But repeated attempts by the pharmaceutical industry to solve the problem with one or another form of "female Viagra" have failed.

My viewpoint: Reviving a mature woman's sex drive requires addressing multiple factors. *These include...*

•**Balancing hormones**—which play a key role in both physical and mental aspects of arousal—particularly during the hormonal changes of perimenopause and menopause.

Treating the pelvic problems of aging, such as vaginal atrophy and dryness, which can cause painful sex.

Here are natural ways to boost libido that consistently work for the mature women in my medical practice. Choose one or two based on your particular needs. If you still have problems, consult a licensed naturopathic physician.

HORMONE HELP

Several herbs and herbal combinations can help balance a mature woman's hormones. *Two of my favorites...*

•**Maca.** This powerful Peruvian herb is a good choice for women going through peri-menopause or menopause because it is rich in plant sterols that balance and strengthen the entire hormonal system. The herb not only increases sex drive but also improves perimeno-pausal and menopausal symptoms such as hot flashes, night sweats and insomnia. Additionally, it supports the adrenal glands, reducing levels of energy-depleting stress hormones.

Typical dose: 1,000 milligrams (mg), twice daily.

•**Two Immortals.** This herbal formula from Traditional Chinese Medicine builds two types of chi, or life-energy—yin (feminine) chi and yang (masculine) chi—thereby boosting a woman's libido, which requires both nurturing (yin) and stimulation (yang).

It also helps to balance hormones and control some symptoms of perimenopause (irregular menstrual bleeding and cramping) and menopause (hot flashes).

Many of my patients take it for six months to a year to rebuild their vitality.

Typical dose: Many companies manufacture the supplement, and dosages vary—follow the dosage recommendation on the label.

SUPER-SEX SUPPLEMENTS

Two nutritional supplements are particularly effective at stimulating sexuality...

•**L-arginine.** This amino acid works by boosting nitric oxide, a compound that promotes blood flow—including blood flow to your genitals.

A study in *Journal of Sex & Marital Therapy* showed that more than 70% of women who took a supplement containing L-arginine (ArginMax for Women) experienced increased sexual desire, more frequent sex and orgasm, enhanced clitoral stimulation, decreased vaginal dryness and improved overall sexual satisfaction.

Typical dose: 3,000 mg daily.

Caution: Talk to your doctor before you take L-arginine, especially if you have low blood pressure, herpes, gastric ulcer, liver disease or kidney disease.

•**PEA (phenylethylamine).** Called the "love supplement," PEA boosts the neurotransmitter dopamine, enhancing feelings of well-being, joy and pleasure.

Typical dose: 60 mg once a day. (Higher doses can cause overstimulation, insomnia or anxiety.)

Caution: Don't take PEA if you're nursing, pregnant or take an MAOI antidepressant medication such as *selegiline* (Eldepryl).

You also can boost PEA by exercising regularly, eating dark chocolate and taking a blue-green algae called spirulina.

APHRODISIACS

Two aphrodisiacs are particularly effective for mature women because—by relaxing your body and improving your mood—they slowly and gently boost your libido.

•**Cordyceps.** This mushroom is considered a potent sexual tonic in Traditional Chinese Medicine. It enhances both yin and yang chi, making it an ideal aphrodisiac for women.

Typical dose: 400 mg, twice daily.

What works best: Pills made by a hot-water extraction process that pulls out the herb's most active constituents, such as the cordyceps supplement from MushroomScience.com.

•**Ginkgo biloba.** Often recommended for memory loss because it improves blood supply to the brain, ginkgo also promotes blood flow to the vulva and vagina. Studies show that it may help restore libido in women taking anti-depressants, which can destroy sex drive.

Typical dose: 40 mg, three times a day. The label should read, "Standardized extract of 24% ginkgo flavonglycosides (or flavone glycosides)."

STATIN WARNING

Cholesterol-lowering statin drugs—taken by millions of older women—can lower libido, probably by damaging mitochondria, energy-generating structures inside cells. If you take a statin and notice a decrease in libido, talk to your doctor about your options.

VAGINAL WEIGHT-TRAINING

The pubococcygeal (PC) muscle—a bowl-shaped "hammock" of pelvic muscle that contracts rhythmically when you have an orgasm and also supports your genital organs and bladder—is crucial to sexual pleasure.

New approach: Using a vaginal weight (a small, round weight inside an oval tube that is inserted into the vagina like a tampon) is the best way to strengthen the PC muscle, enhancing erotic sensation and sexual response.

What to do: To start, insert the tube for one to five minutes, twice daily, squeezing your PC muscle repeatedly to hold the tube in place. You can do this standing or lying down. Gradually work up to 20 minutes, twice daily, using progressively heavier weights. Do this for three months. You can order a set of vaginal weights at *Vagacare.com*.

Cost: About $30.

Other benefits: Regular use of vaginal weights can help prevent and treat urinary incontinence and prevent prolapse of the bladder or uterus.

VAGINAL DRYNESS AND PAINFUL INTERCOURSE

Enjoyable sex requires vaginal tissue that is healthy and well-hydrated. But the midlife drop in estrogen levels causes a decrease of blood flow to the vagina, which can lead to vaginal atrophy and dryness. *A simple remedy…*

• **Vitamin E.** The unique lubricating properties of vitamin E make it especially effective.

What to do: Pierce a soft 400 IU vitamin E gel capsule with a pin, squeeze the oil onto your finger, and apply it to the outside of the vagina and inside about an inch. Or use a vitamin E vaginal suppository. (I recommend the product from Earth's Botanical Harvest, available online.) Apply the gel or insert the suppository nightly at bedtime for at least two weeks. Taper use to three times a week.

Great Sex, Naturally— Men: The Secret to Better Erections

Steven Lamm, MD, a practicing internist, faculty member at New York University School of Medicine and director of Men's Health for the NYU Medical Center, both in New York City. He is author of *The Hardness Factor: How to Achieve Your Best Health and Fitness At Any Age.* His most recent book is *No Guts, No Glory.* DrSteven Lamm.com

I f you're like most middle-aged and older men, you want better erections—erections that are reliable and hard. *But better sex is only one of the benefits of better erections…*

Surprising fact: A man's erection is an important barometer of his health. Erectile dysfunction (ED)—when a man can't get or keep an erection firm enough for sexual intercourse—often is an early warning sign of heart disease. An erection requires healthy blood vessels, nerves and hormones.

Important scientific evidence: A seven-year study of more than 4,000 middle-aged and older men, published in *The Journal of the American Medical Association,* showed that those who had ED at the beginning of the study or developed it during the study had a 45% higher risk of developing heart disease.

Unfortunately, ED affects roughly half of American men over age 60 (and many younger men)—most of whom have cardiovascular disease or one or more risk factors for developing it, such as high cholesterol, high blood pressure, insulin resistance, diabetes or obesity.

Of course, you can take an ED drug (such as Viagra, Cialis or Levitra) for the problem. But that won't take care of the underlying health issues. Plus, no man wants to be dependent on ED drugs...they're not without risk (blindness is a rare but possible side effect)...and they don't always work.

Here's what you need to know to preserve or restore your erections—and the health of your body—naturally...

●**Exercise**

Erections owe most of their hardness to nitric oxide, a molecule that signals blood vessels to relax, allowing blood to enter and pool in the penis. The body's most effective way of stimulating nitric oxide formation is exercise—even mild exercise, such as walking.

Scientific evidence: In a study of 180 men ages 40 to 70, published in *International Journal of Impotence Research*, those who were sedentary were 10 times more likely to develop ED than those who were physically active.

My recommendation: 10,000 steps a day, which you can achieve through everyday physical activity (typically 4,000 to 5,000 steps) and a brisk walk of 4,000 to 6,000 steps (about two to three miles, or 30 to 45 minutes).

Start with 5,000 steps daily for one week. Increase to 6,000 steps daily the second week... and to 7,000 the third week...until you reach 10,000. Maintain that level. You can find an accurate pedometer—typically at a cost of $20 to $30—at your local sporting-goods store or on the Internet at *www.DigiWalker.com.*

ERECTION-ENHANCING FOODS

Your sexual performance is greatly impacted by the foods you eat. *My recommendations...*

●**Reduce the fats in your diet.** Fatty foods lead to clogged arteries, which prevent blood flow from reaching the penis. Cut back on saturated fats such as egg yolks, butter, cream, fatty red meats and palm oil.

●**Eat more fruits and vegetables.** They reduce cholesterol and improve blood flow to the penis.

●**Eat whole grains, nuts and seeds.** They provide an important basis for cardiovascular and penile health.

●**Spice up your foods.** Chili peppers stimulate the nervous system, helping with sexual arousal. Ginger has long been considered a

sexual stimulant and an overall tonic for general health.

BEST SUPPLEMENTS

Several supplements can help restore erections...

●**L-arginine and Pycnogenol.** The amino acid L-arginine (found in meat, whole grains, fish, nuts and milk) is converted to nitric oxide in the body. But most men don't get enough in their diets, so I often recommend an L-arginine supplement.*

L-arginine works best when combined with Pycnogenol, a patented amalgam of more than three dozen antioxidants extracted from the bark of the French pine tree. Together, the supplement allows for better nitric oxide production and utilization.

Scientific research: In a study of men with mild-to-moderate ED, published in Phytotherapy Research, taking a supplement with L-arginine and Pycnogenol for eight weeks improved erections and satisfaction with sex.

Typical dose: A daily dose of the supplement Prelox Blue, which contains a blend of Pycnogenol and L-arginine.

●**Omega-3 fatty acids (fish oil).** Found in oily fish such as salmon and sardines, omega-3s can reduce plaque inside artery walls... decrease blood clotting...lower triglyceride (blood fat) levels...and decrease both blood pressure and blood vessel inflammation. Omega-3s are the nutritional building blocks of heart and penis health.

Typical dose: 2,000 milligrams (mg) daily, taken with a meal.

●**Horny goat weed (Epimedium sagittatum).** This Chinese herb perks up sexual desire.

Scientific evidence: I conducted two studies on Exotica H-G-W, a brand of horny goat weed. The first study showed that the supplement enhanced sexual satisfaction in three out of five men. The second study—in which men took horny goat weed capsules one hour before sexual activity—resulted in a signifi-

*Caution: Talk to your doctor before taking L-arginine, especially if you have low blood pressure, herpes, gastric ulcer, liver disease or kidney disease.

cant increase in hardness in two-thirds of the participants.

Typical dose: Two capsules daily, totaling 500 mg of horny goat weed. My patients take it for six weeks and then start to taper off. You can use it intermittently after that.

TESTOSTERONE SELF-CARE

Testosterone—the predominantly male hormone that helps drive sexual desire and performance—declines with age. But most of that decline is caused by lifestyle—poor sleep, relentless stress and belly fat. *My recommendations...*

•**Sleep seven to eight hours a night.** Going to bed at the same time every night (say, 11:00 pm) and getting up at the same time every morning (say, 6:30 am) is one of the best habits for deep, refreshing sleep.

•**Add strength-training to your routine.** Whether it's in the gym or at home with resistance bands, building and maintaining muscle are key to producing plenty of testosterone.

•**Breathe.** Take a few slow, deep breaths a few times a day every single day—it does wonders for relieving tension and anxiety.

VISUALIZE FOR SEX SUCCESS

How do you prepare for an upcoming sexual encounter, especially if you didn't do so well in a previous effort and don't feel confident?

Sex is a physical act—and just as athletes practice visualization techniques so they can perform optimally, you can use the same techniques to build confidence in your bedroom "performance."

First, relax—lie on your back on a mat or a rug with your arms at your sides and take a deep breath. Hold it for a moment, then exhale. Lie still, and continue breathing slowly.

Once you are relaxed, picture yourself about to have sex. Patiently go through the step-by-step sequence of events. Imagine every aspect of the session, including the sights, sounds and smells associated with sex. Try to rehearse the action in your mind just as you would actually perform it. It's all about mental practice. When the time comes for the actual moment, your confidence will be higher.

The Truth About Sexual-Enhancement Herbs For Men

Laurie Steelsmith, ND, LAc, licensed naturopathic physician and acupuncturist in private practice in Honolulu. Dr. Steelsmith is coauthor, with her husband Alex Steelsmith, of *Great Sex, Naturally: Every Woman's Guide to Enhancing Her Sexuality Through the Secrets of Natural Medicine.* DrLaurieSteelsmith.com

Herbal supplements might seem like a good idea if you are a man who is having "trouble" in the bedroom. They're easy to buy—locally or online—and you don't have to discuss this embarrassing problem with your doctor.

Or maybe you think these natural products are safer than Viagra or other pharmaceuticals and may, in fact, have health benefits that go beyond improving your sex life.

But...some of the most common herbs for male sexual enhancement have been bashed by the medical establishment—yohimbe, maca, horny goat weed and even ginkgo biloba.

How much weight should you give that news? First, let's examine what's being said about male sexual-enhancement herbs. Then let naturopathic sex-health and Traditional Chinese Medicine expert Laurie Steelsmith, ND, LAc, reveal the real dos, don'ts and dangers of these herbs.

THE DANGER OF SEXY SUPPLEMENTS

A recent article by a team of British and Italian researchers said that the business of selling herbal supplements for male sexual enhancement—or dysfunction—is a major health hazard. Because these supplements are marketed as "natural," many consumers assume that they are safe. In fact, they can cause serious side effects in some users.

In their exposé, the researchers focused on supplements that contained four herbs commonly used to treat male sexual dysfunction—yohimbe, maca, horny goat weed and ginkgo biloba. In brief, they concluded that all of these herbs were linked to dangerous side effects, including cardiovascular problems, mood swings, anxiety, hallucinations and addictive behavior.

Dr. Steelsmith, however, believes that these researchers have been overly harsh. "They are making herbs, such as ginkgo, out to be radical villains, which they are not," she said, adding that ginkgo and maca have long-term safety records. She also said that horny goat weed is safe when used according to the principles of Traditional Chinese Medicine. But she agreed that the researchers made some good points about yohimbe, which can cause high blood pressure, dangerously low blood pressure, increased heart rate and palpitations, breathing difficulties, headaches and anxiety among other symptoms. "It is a potentially dangerous herb. Unlike the other herbs discussed, I don't think it should be sold over the counter, but certain formulations of the herb can be used with medical supervision," she said.

PRACTICE "SAFE SEX SUPPLEMENTS"

Most common sex-enhancement herbs are safe and effective when used correctly, said Dr. Steelsmith, who is the coauthor of the book *Great Sex, Naturally*. Rather than self-treating, it is best to consult a naturopathic doctor or similarly trained professional who can properly diagnose your health concern and treat you with specially compounded herbal extracts and extracts from high-quality professional-grade manufacturers. *Here are her expert thoughts on the sex-boosting herbs mentioned in the British-Italian study…*

• **Yohimbe.** Rather than use over-the-counter extracts, always consult a naturopathic doctor if you want to try yohimbe. Dr. Steelsmith reserves such treatment for patients who are in good health but have erectile dysfunction that does not respond to other less potentially toxic remedies. If yohimbe is right for you, a naturopath will treat you with a prescription form of the herb called alpha yohimbine HCl, said Dr. Steelsmith. The naturopath will monitor you while you take yohimbe to make sure that the dosage is optimal and side effects are kept at bay. Men with kidney problems or psychological issues should not take or be treated with this herb.

• **Horny goat weed.** This herb is useful for men who have decreased libido, a slow metabolism and chronically cold hands and feet. In Traditional Chinese Medicine, horny goat weed is never prescribed on its own but rather in combination with herbs that support its ability to boost sexual energy while preventing side effects of overstimulation, said Dr. Steelsmith. Because horny goat weed can act as a stimulant, it is not for you if you suffer from insomnia or anxiety symptoms. Dr. Steelsmith also does not recommend it's use in people who are on are on blood-thinning medications.

Important: Make sure that the herbal extract prescribed by the naturopath is a standardized extract that contains at least 20% of the active compound icariin.

• **Maca.** This Peruvian herb, traditionally used to increase male sexual potency and endurance, enhances male fertility, said Dr. Steelsmith. It increases sperm production and renders those critters into super-triathlete swimmers (it keeps them strongly mobile, that is). So if a man is ready to start a family, Dr. Steelsmith often prescribes maca. It is generally safe, but be aware that it can increase blood pressure, an issue that you should discuss with the naturopath, especially if you already have high blood pressure.

• **Ginkgo biloba.** Besides boosting memory and cognitive function, ginkgo biloba can boost libido and enhance sexual performance. It is especially useful in both men as well as women who are suffering sexual dysfunction as a side effect of antidepressant medication, said Dr. Steelsmith. A word of caution, though…ginkgo is a natural blood thinner and can interact with blood-thinning drugs as well as other drugs that are broken down by the liver (and most are)—so if you are on a blood thinner or any other type of medication or supplement, ginkgo biloba may not be the right herb for you. This aside, Dr. Steelsmith said that it is safe at the dosages that naturopaths use to treat erectile dysfunction. The product prescribed should be a standardized extract of 24% ginkgo flavone glycosides.

Beside these herbs mentioned in the alarming Brit-Italian study, Dr. Steelsmith treats patients with *Tribulus terrestris*, which acts similarly to DHEA, an essential building block of estrogen and testosterone that can help keep you young and fit. The extract should contain

45% of the active ingredient protodioscin. It is especially useful in men whose low sex drive is attributed to low testosterone, said Dr. Steelsmith. The herb may support testosterone production. Dr. Steelsmith cautioned that lithium and diabetes drugs can interact with this herb, so anyone taking those medications is not a candidate for use of this herb.

MORE THAN JUST SEX

Before grabbing any herb or drug to fix a sexual-performance problem, it's wise to reflect on the underlying cause of the problem and make the necessary lifestyle changes, said Dr. Steelsmith. Are you stressed or sleep-deprived? Anxious or depressed? Is a physical health condition getting in the way of good sex? Treating the root cause may solve your sexual dysfunction without any other measures.

Dangerous Overtreatment of Low Testosterone: What You Can Do Naturally

Glenn R. Cunningham, MD, professor of medicine and molecular and cell biology, Baylor College of Medicine, and endocrinologist, St. Luke's Episcopal Hospital, both in Houston.

J. Bradley Layton, PhD, postdoctoral researcher, department of epidemiology, University of North Carolina, Chapel Hill, and leader of a study on testosterone testing and treatment published in *Journal of Clinical Endocrinology and Metabolism*.

Have you seen the TV commercials targeting men who are "feeling down"... seem like "shadows of their former selves"...and have "lost their appetite for romance"? The voice-over suggests that a hormone problem may be causing their symptoms, then routes viewers' attention to a website that markets testosterone-replacement therapy.

The ads are part of a so-called disease-awareness campaign, with the condition in question being low testosterone (aka low T)...and the implied solution being testosterone therapy.

Problem: This treatment may increase the risk of suffering a heart attack or dying! De-

spite the potential dangers, use of the treatment has quadrupled in the US over the course of a decade. In some cases, this therapy is being prescribed for men who don't need it—including those whose testosterone levels are normal. Why this surge in usage? In part, because testosterone therapy is big business—a whopping $1.6 billion-per-year business.

Still, we shouldn't be too quick to slam the whole idea of testosterone therapy—because some men really do require and benefit from the treatment...and because the studies showing risks are contradicted by other studies suggesting that testosterone therapy is safe.

Clearly, this is not a settled topic, and misimpression and misinformation abound. So to help readers make sense of it all, we spoke to two experts on the subject. *Here's what you should know...*

JUST WHAT IS LOW T?

Low testosterone is sometimes a sign of hypogonadism, a syndrome caused by a glitch with one of three glands that normally work together—the pituitary, the hypothalamus and the testes. When something goes awry within this system, the testes end up producing too little testosterone (and fewer sperm).

Symptoms: Hypogonadism can lead to loss of height, body hair and muscle mass...low-trauma bone fractures (bones that fracture easily)...hot flashes and sweats...breast tissue development...and fertility problems. Hypogonadism also causes less specific symptoms—fatigue, sleep disturbances, low libido, reduced strength, poor concentration, depression—though, of course, these vague symptoms can result from other health problems as well.

However, low testosterone by itself does not signal hypogonadism. Especially in the absence of clear symptoms, a reduced testosterone level does not necessarily indicate a problem that needs treatment.

How low is too low? Unfortunately, there is no clear answer to that question. One reason for the current overtreatment of low T is that it's not easy to draw a line between normal testosterone levels and abnormally low levels. *Here's why...*

•**The lower limit of the normal range varies depending on whom you ask.** Some experts give a cutoff of 200 nanograms of testosterone per deciliter (ng/dL) of blood, while others define low T as anything below 300 ng/dL or even 350 ng/dL.

However "normal" is defined, those numbers were established by looking at healthy young men—so they aren't necessarily applicable to older men. Testosterone levels typically do fall with age, declining by about 1% to 2% per year beginning in men's 40s or 50s. By the time men are in their 60s, one-fifth have testosterone levels that some doctors would consider low…by their 80s, about one-half of men have testosterone levels that some would call low. The fact that older men are more likely than younger ones to have chronic medical conditions that affect hormone levels makes it more difficult to pinpoint how much of the testosterone decline is attributable to normal aging.

•**Testosterone tests are not standardized.** For one thing, there are various types of tests. Some measure total testosterone…others measure what's called free (unbound) testosterone, which is a mere fraction of the total…still others measure bioavailable testosterone, which also is less than the total. A doctor who's not well-versed in the differences could wrongly interpret the numbers that these different tests yield. Furthermore, lab results don't always agree—so two different labs (even careful labs) can come up with two very different numbers.

A man's testosterone level fluctuates throughout the day, with the highest reading in the morning, so his test results depend in part on the time of day at which his blood was drawn. Even among healthy young men, for instance, 15% will have a testosterone reading that drops below the normal range at some point in a 24-hour period. Often these daily fluctuations are not taken into consideration when interpreting test results.

One man's low is not necessarily the same as another man's because the level at which symptoms appear varies widely. And the presence or absence of symptoms makes a big difference (or at least it should make a big difference, as we'll discuss in a moment) in the decision about whether or not to treat low T.

INCREASED TESTING, INCREASED TREATMENT

Despite the lack of any agreed-upon definition of testosterone deficiency, testosterone testing and replacement therapy have become very popular in the US…in some cases, even among men who probably don't need it.

For instance, a study led by epidemiologist J. Bradley Layton, PhD, of the University of North Carolina at Chapel Hill, found that testosterone testing increased 329% from 2000 to 2010—an increase that researchers attributed in part to heavy direct-to-consumer marketing (such as those TV ads encouraging men to get their mojo back).

Disturbingly, among the American men who started on testosterone replacement, pretreatment testing showed that about 20% already had normal or high testosterone levels…and 40% started treatment without having been recently tested at all!

QUESTIONS ABOUT SAFETY

Dr. Layton's study is not the first to sound alarms about testosterone therapy.

For instance: In one observational study of veterans with low testosterone, those who started replacement therapy were 30% more likely to have a heart attack or stroke or to die from any cause during the study period. In another observational study, in the 90 days after starting testosterone therapy, nonfatal heart attack risk rose 36% overall…more than doubled for men age 65 and up…and nearly tripled for men under age 65 who had a history of heart disease. And one clinical trial of older men was stopped early when it became obvious that the men on testosterone therapy had a significantly higher risk for heart attack or irregular heart rhythm than the participants taking a placebo.

However, while the results of the above studies are worrisome, they don't tell the whole story. For one thing, it's important to note that there's considerable data showing that low testosterone itself is associated with increased cardiovascular and mortality risks, according to Glenn R. Cunningham, MD, an endocrinologist at Baylor College of Medicine in Houston. Dr. Cunningham was a member of a task force that wrote the 2010 guidelines on testing and treating testosterone deficiency for the Endocrine Society, a professional organization devoted to research on hormones and the clinical practice of endocrinology.

Also, the studies cited above have limitations. In the veterans study, the analysis of the data may have been flawed, Dr. Cunningham said—and a different veterans' study showed that testosterone therapy was associated with a lower risk of dying. Also, a meta-analysis of about 50 small observational studies did not find an increase in cardiovascular events or death. And in the clinical trial cited above, the testosterone dosage was higher than is normally prescribed—whereas in a large European study that used more typical dosages, treatment did not increase cardiovascular risk.

Bottom line: "At this point, we do not know if there is danger of increased cardiovascular events associated with testosterone treatment—and we need a very rigorous, placebo-controlled trial, following at least 6,000 men for at least five years, to find out," Dr. Cunningham said.

WHAT MEN CONSIDERING TREATMENT CAN DO

If you are concerned about possible low T, the first step is to visit your doctor and discuss your symptoms. If you have any of the more specific signs that suggest hypogonadism (such as loss of height, hot flashes or breast tissue development or a history of low-trauma bone fractures), testing is definitely warranted, Dr. Cunningham said. With the more vague symptoms (decreased energy, increased body fat, low libido, concentration or mood problems), testosterone testing may be considered—though it's also important to rule out other conditions that could underlie such symptoms.

•**Testing is not a one-shot deal**—because up to 30% of men who initially have a low testosterone measurement have a normal level on their next test without any therapy. Dr. Cunningham stressed that if a second test, done at least a few days later, also shows a low testosterone level, it's important to keep digging for more information. "More sophisticated lab tests can tell if the problem is originating in the testes or in either the pituitary gland or

hypothalamus. Also, because the protein that carries testosterone in the blood is reduced in overweight and obese men, such patients may need special tests to uncover their true testosterone levels," he said.

It's also important to explore whether low testosterone itself actually is causing the symptoms…or whether, instead, some other underlying problem is causing the symptoms and affecting testosterone levels. Low testosterone can be the result of depression, stress, sleep apnea, eating disorders, pituitary tumors, liver or kidney abnormalities, and many other systemic illnesses. In such cases, Dr. Cunningham said, "Treatment of the associated medical problem may improve testosterone levels. If it does not, testosterone therapy may be helpful."

The Endocrine Society's guidelines suggest treating low testosterone only when symptoms are present and when testing shows unequivocally low testosterone levels. Even then, it's essential to weigh the benefits against the risks while taking overall health status into consideration. Testosterone therapy may be inadvisable for a man with heart disease…uncontrolled sleep apnea, which can worsen with testosterone therapy…a history of blood clots, because testosterone therapy can increase clotting…or a high hematocrit (a measure of red blood cell concentration), which may increase further if testosterone is given, elevating heart attack risk. Some doctors also advise against testosterone therapy for men who have been treated for prostate cancer, though others say that it's OK.

NATURAL WAYS TO BOOST TESTOSTERONE

Before you resort to hormone therapy, it's also wise to talk with your doctor about safe, natural ways to increase testosterone levels. *It often helps to…*

•**Lose excess weight.** One 2012 study found that obese men can increase their testosterone levels by 15% by shedding just 17 pounds.

•**Maintain a healthful diet that includes plenty of vegetables,** fruits, whole grains, legumes and monounsaturated fats…limits processed carbohydrates, such as sugar and white flour…and emphasizes organic food (since estrogen-like pesticides can stymie testosterone).

• **Get your vitamin D level tested**—and if it is low, ask your doctor about taking daily supplements of vitamin D-3.

• **Get regular exercise,** including weight lifting and interval training (for instance, exercise to maximum capacity for one minute… slow down until normal breathing is restored, usually about one minute…then repeat that two-part cycle for 20 minutes).

• **Limit alcohol to no more than two drinks a day…don't smoke…manage stress…and get adequate sleep.**

Remember: Such healthy lifestyle practices can go a long way toward normalizing testosterone levels—without the risks that go along with testosterone-replacement therapy.

Sexy Smoothies and More

Mark A. Moyad, MD, MPH, the Jenkins/Pokempner Director of Preventive & Alternative Medicine in the department of urology at the University of Michigan Medical Center in Ann Arbor. Dr. Moyad, who specializes in nondrug medicinal therapies, is the lead author of more than 150 medical articles and 11 books, including *The Supplement Handbook.* He created the recipes in this article with his wife, Mia Moyad.

Everybody knows about the "little blue pill" (also known as Viagra). It and similar drugs help men perform sexually by opening up and relaxing blood vessels in the penis. But some men suffer headaches, stomach upset and other side effects. And for women? Addyi (*flibanserin*), the "little pink pill" created to boost female libido, turns out to be a poor performer with its own set of side effects.

A safe option: Many fruits and vegetables can improve sexual functioning in much the same way that prescription medications do.

Hard to believe? It's true. These foods, including bananas, kale and watermelon, are rich in inorganic compounds, such as nitrate and nitrite, and other compounds that play a key role in men's—and women's—sexual arousal, performance and response. These compounds are such powerhouses because they have the ability to increase levels of nitric oxide (NO)—a molecule that dilates blood vessels and increases blood flow to many organs, including the sexual organs.

Bonus: NO's beneficial effect on blood vessels also helps reduce heart disease risk by lowering blood pressure. Tasty recipes to improve your sex life—and heart health…*

SEXY SMOOTHIE

Blend (start on "low" and increase to "high"): One-half cup of ice…one cup of unsweetened coconut water…one-half cup of shredded kale…one-half frozen banana…one-half cup of your favorite frozen berries (for some extra sweetness, if desired)…one to two pitted prunes…plus one tablespoon of L-citrulline (an amino acid that creates NO) or dried Panax ginseng powder (an herb that promotes sexual desire).

Why it works: Bananas are a great source of nitrate and nitrite. Coconut water, bananas and kale are rich sources of blood pressure–lowering potassium…and prunes deliver fiber, which helps control blood sugar—important for heart health and blood pressure control.

• **L-citrulline is the closest thing there is to an over-the-counter**

• **Viagra.** It's available as a powder or in capsule form (empty out two or three capsules to get 1,000 mg to 1,500 mg of powder…or simply swallow them with your smoothie).

Good product: Source Naturals' L-Citrulline powder, *VitaminShoppe.com.*

• **Red Panax ginseng** has been found in research to significantly improve sexual arousal in menopausal women. Select a brand with at least 8% ginsenosides (the main active components of Panax ginseng).

Good product: NuSci Panax Ginseng Extract Powder, Standardized 10% Ginsenosides, *Amazon.com.*

Note: Breast cancer patients should not use ginseng products.

*Some ingredients in these recipes may interact with certain medications—such as *warfarin* (Coumadin) and blood pressure or erectile dysfunction drugs. Consult your doctor.

HIGH-OCTANE SMOOTHIE

Blend (Start on "low" and increase to "high"): One cup of ice…one cup of almond milk…two tablespoons of natural, no-sugar-added peanut butter…one-half frozen banana…one-half-inch jalapeño or a dash of cayenne pepper…one teaspoon of coconut or palm oil…and one tablespoon of cacao powder.

Why it works: This smoothie lifts your energy levels—crucial for a good sex life. Peanut butter is a stellar source of protein, which helps maintain metabolism and muscle function. If you don't like peanut butter, try another nut butter—or a scoop of flavored protein powder.

Good product: Jay Robb Whey Protein Powder, *GNC.com.*

Capsaicin, the compound responsible for the fiery heat of jalapeño and cayenne pepper, increases NO and blood flow throughout the body. Coconut and palm oils provide a type of healthful fat that is easily used by the body for energy. Cacao contains *anandamide*, a feel-good neurotransmitter, and just enough caffeine for a little natural lift.

WATERMELON SANGRIA

Combine: One bottle of red wine with a sliced orange, lemon and lime, plus two cups of club soda. Then add one cup of watermelon juice (buy it online or make your own) and one cup of shaved watermelon rind (shave the white part of the rind on the inside of the watermelon).

Why it works: This summer cocktail features heart-healthy red wine. What makes this recipe different is the L-citrulline (found in watermelon juice and rind), which improves NO production. The alcohol will lower inhibitions to help put you in the mood for sex. But don't have more than two four- to six-ounce glasses. Too much will steal your mojo!

The Sexiest Scent May Already Be Your Perfume…or Cologne

Study titled, "The smelling of Hedione results in sex-differentiated human brain activity" by researchers in the department of cell physiology at Ruhr University in Bochum, and in the departments of neuroradiology and otorhinolaryngology at Technische Universität in Dresden, both in Germany, published in *NeuroImage.*

When the subject is romance, the nose knows. For years, scientists have been debating whether certain scents play a role in human sexual attraction. Now researchers in Germany have found that humans do respond strongly to a specific fragrance—in ways that could ignite a woman's sex drive.

What's more, you may already be wearing this particular floral jasmine-magnolia ingredient. It's found in many high-end perfumes and men's fragrances.

Remember this ingredient name—hedione. It comes from the Greek word for pleasure.

ON THE TRAIL OF A HUMAN PHEROMONE

For decades, scientists have debated whether there are human pheromones. In animals, pheromones are chemicals that are released by individuals in a species to influence the sexual behavior of other members of the same species in predictable ways. When the female silkworm releases the molecule *bombykol*, for example, male silkworms drop everything and come hither.

We humans are more complex. Certainly, how we smell to each other affects our hormones, which may influence behavior, sexual and otherwise. For example, the odor of perspiration plays a role in the synchronization of the menstrual cycles of women who live or work together. In men, the scent of a T-shirt worn by an ovulating woman leads to testosterone levels going up, while the scent of a woman's tears of sadness causes testosterone levels to drop. Human odors are linked with behaviors as diverse as the fear response and mother/baby bonding.

The question, though, is whether specific molecules elicit these specific responses, especially sexual. That is, are there really human pheromones?

The authors of the new study out of Germany think the answer is…yes.

A FLORAL TURN-ON FOR WOMEN

In the German study, researchers from Ruhr University in Bochum and their colleagues at the Technische Universität in Dresden examined how receptors in the nasal cavity and certain areas of the human brain responded when 17 healthy male and female volunteers smelled the scent of hedione (chemical name *methyl dihydrojasmonate*), a compound first synthesized in the 1960s by a chemist seeking to reproduce the intoxicating scent of jasmine. The researchers then compared the results with what happened when the same participants smelled a common floral fragrance, phenylethyl alcohol, which smells like rose water.

What they found is that the hedione scent activated the vomeronasal receptor (VN1R) that humans have in their noses. This is the organ that acts as a pheromone receptor in other mammals but hasn't been shown to be active in humans—until now. Just as importantly, using functional magnetic resonance imaging (fMRI), the researchers also found that smelling hedione activated areas in the brain's limbic system, which is associated with emotions, memory and motivation, significantly more strongly than phenylethyl alcohol did.

What's more, hedione activated a specific region in the hypothalamus that's associated with the release of sex hormones. The effect was much stronger in women than in men, and the women in the study rated the fragrance as "significantly more intense" than the men did.

In other words, it appears that this scent may be the first to be discovered that directly turns women on. Of course, there needs to be more research. This study wasn't designed to measure actual hormonal changes, so whether hedione directly affects hormones will have to wait for the next study.

Here's a suggestion for the researchers next time: Ask the women whether smelling the fragrance makes them feel sexier.

WHAT STEVE McQUEEN KNEW

In the meantime, if you want to help a woman you love get in the mood, you might look to the example of the 1960s' movie actor Steve McQueen. He was known to wear Dior's Eau Savage, a cologne for men, introduced in 1966, that was the first product to contain hedione. It's still available after all these years. Hedione is also an ingredient in the colognes cK One by Calvin Klein, Acqua di Giò by Giorgio Armani, and Voyage d'Hermes Parfum for men and women by Hermes.

Hedione is also in some women's perfumes, including Diorella from Dior, First by Van Cleef & Arpels, Chanel No. 19 (by Chanel of course), Blush by Marc Jacobs, and L'Eau d'Issey by Issey Miyake. Like to make your own perfume or cologne? You can buy pure hedione directly from perfume ingredient supply companies such as *CreatingPerfume.com*. You may even want to add some to an existing perfume or cologne—the amount that professionals include ranges from just a few percent up to 35% by volume.

We're already brainstorming names for our own concoction.

When Sex = Happiness

How often should you have sex? Studies of more than 30,000 people show that couples who make love once a week report the highest level of happiness—more than those who have sex less frequently but no less than those who exceed a weekly tryst.

Explanation: Weekly sex is optimal to maintain an intimate connection between partners with busy lives.

Amy Muise, PhD, postdoctoral fellow, University of Toronto, Ontario, Canada.